Miranda Mattig Kumar

Heal Your
Body and Mind

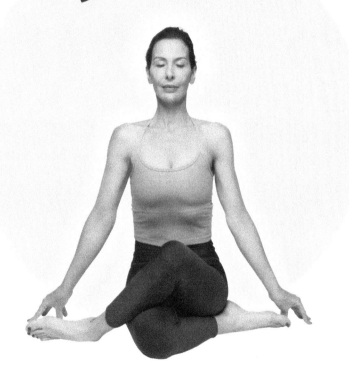

With Yin Yoga

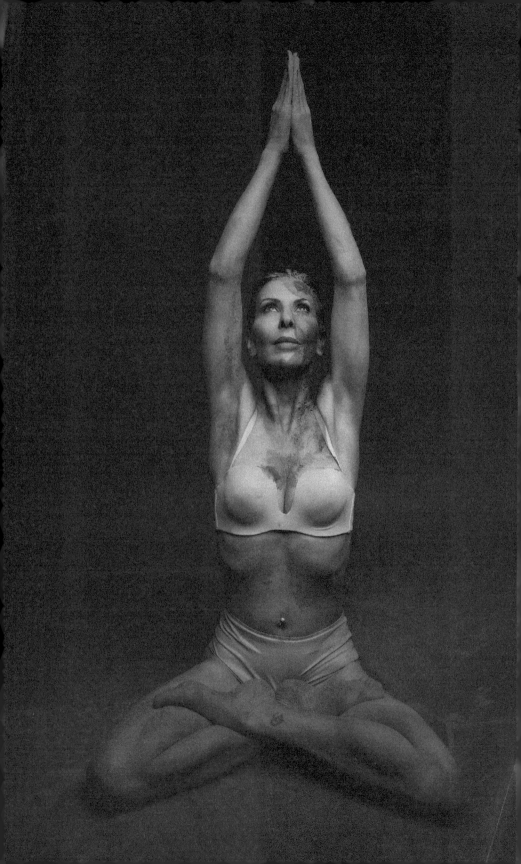

Quadrant Books

First published in 2023 by Quadrant Books

Suite 2, Top Floor, 7 Dyer Street, Cirencester, Gloucestershire, GL7 2PF

Heal Your Body and Mind with Yin Yoga
Paperback ISBN 978-1-7398645-4-5

Design by Ray Lipscombe, Cirencester
Printed and bound in Great Britain

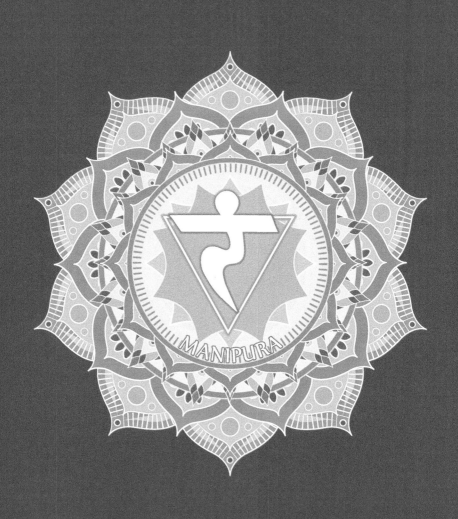

Contents

6 The Energy System: the Chakras

7 How The Meridians Are Stimulated by the Practice of Yin?

8 Yin Yoga Poses

This book is much more than printed words on paper. Just scan one of the QR codes with your tablet, Android or iPhone and you'll be taken straight to a video which will provide an introduction to the benefits of Yin Yoga. If your device isn't QR scan enabled, just download the videos free from Google Play.

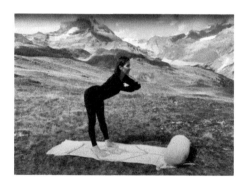

1. Yin session: this session targets the stretching of the fascia in your posterior muscles groups. You will experience looser hamstrings and hips, which will provide you with a feeling of being able to move freer and being lighter.

2. Yin for a healthy back - You will find Yin yoga postures which relieve your back pain. By stretching your hamstrings, hips and piriformis you will release the tension in your lower back.

3. Yin - Heart opening practice : This Yin Yoga session will help you improve your posture by stretching your chest muscles, which improves the alignment of your ears, shoulders, hips and heels.

4. Yin - Hip opening session: In this Yin yoga session you will work on getting more mobility and flexibility in your hips. Releasing this tension will give you a feeling of more stability and being grounded.

Foreword

My name is Miranda Mattig Kumar. I am a certified yoga therapist with a Swiss Federal diploma and in this book I would like to share what I have learned by practising yoga for over 25 year

If you know a bit about this philosophy, you know it is not gymnastics, nor a sport, but a way of living.

The beauty of yoga is that it is accessible to everyone with all its physical, emotional, and spiritual aspects. I will lead you to a discovery of Yin Yoga, its anatomical basis, the meridians, and chakras, to develop a greater knowledge of your body and energy centers.

You will learn to change the practice according to your needs. You can use accessories to be more comfortable in the poses. To get there, I have summarized the physiology of the human body to explain the relevant parts, so you have a better understanding of how your system functions. You will understand what a trendy phenomenon the fascia, is and how stretching them will miraculously eliminate your physical tension.

You will find the definition of various pathologies, as well as the poses proven to treat them efficiently. And I dare to go further! Since the human being is a whole, I invite you to analyze the emotional sources of those ailments. You will see what the energy centers are and think about their connection to your physical and emotional symptoms, so you can then treat them.

In yoga philosophy, we talk about Prana, or Chi, breathing and energy, always present. The deepening of this knowledge makes you aware of the importance of noticing them.

Personally, I began during my teenage years, by reading about meditation and personal development, focusing especially on creative visualization. I would like to share this with you regarding Yin Yoga, and the emotional and symbolic aspects of the various pathologies. You quickly realize that the body, spirit, and mind form a connected, interdependent unity. Your initial motivation might be physical, but after a short while, you will feel there is another dimension to this practice.

My complicated teenage years made me grow. I already felt back then that seeing things clearly was difficult, but it was the only way to go forward on my personal path. The mental, spiritual, and physical connections were already present. Each time I was sick, I knew very well that my resilience was low because negative circumstances were piling up; they manifested physically because I was ignoring them. I needed to solve them to heal!

A bit later, when I was about 19 and in Maryland (USA) at the dance academy, I started my physical practice of yoga poses to gain flexibility. It calmed me, and although I knew nothing about the philosophy of yoga, I felt it went beyond a simple physical practice. At 22, I went to Galicia, Spain, for my first training in Hatha Yoga. I continued with Ashtanga Yoga, a more dynamic style, and discovered my strong passion for this practice.

Although I felt weak and not flexible enough, I felt a deep calm during the final relaxation, Savasana, that I had never felt before.

I started to practice every day, which refocused me and made me feel good.

My thirst for adventure brought me to study and work in Miami, Montréal, Lugano, Barcelona, Sydney, and Geneva. Since I always went alone, I was faced with myself. I wanted to be guided, and I referred to books to find tips and inspiration. Intuition, positive thinking, the law of attraction, the let-go principle. They were all part of that and gave me the strength and courage to continue along my path.

I finally understood that speaking seven languages and changing countries yearly were just escape routes from facing reality. Since 2005, I have been practicing in Geneva, where I have created many training programs for yoga of 200 and 300 hours, Pilates, and therapeutic yoga. I learn and progress with my students and consider myself fortunate to live my passion.

Dynamic yoga practice was a passion of mine. However, as the years passed, I realized that some of my clients had other needs which it did not match. I started including accessories like a chair, a wall, a belt, and blocks—they were a hit!

When I started to write my professional essay for my Federal Diploma of Therapeutic Yoga, I realized how therapeutic Yin Yoga is. It is very moving that its benefits are obvious to clients with reduced mobility and pathologies which do not allow them to follow a more rigorous practice. I had an efficient and simple flexibility training I could use with my senior citizens, who were thrilled and amazed at their progress. Those results were also beneficial to my younger, more dynamic clients. Finding the balance between do and be, Yin and Yang, and be active and at rest, sets a condition for optimal health.

I reached the conclusion that Yin Yoga, along with meditation, creative visualization, and the fulfillment and deepening of what I have done so far, has brought my clients to a place of deep balance.

I would like you to benefit from those experiences and want to help you put in place a practice that meets your needs.

I must admit that, at the beginning, I had problems in letting go and remaining focused. It was not my habit to remain in sitting positions that long, and there was a counter-nature aspect to it. Calming my head and my thoughts without rigorous practice was a genuine challenge. I needed time to assimilate all the benefits of this incredible practice. I decided to integrate Yin into my personal practice to create harmony in my life and find that state of peace again. I learned that by starting with a Yang Practice, a dynamic one, I can chase out the negative energy and then be ready for the softer aspects of Yin.

I hope you can keep your mind open to integrate the benefits of Yin and go beyond the moments of potential doubt to create interior harmony for yourself.

Note from the author

With Yin Yoga, I discovered something that touched me profoundly. I had always believed in emotional symptoms, as well as the connection between mind, body, and spirit.

In my therapeutic practice, I often see clients progressing on their self-healing path by aligning the physical, psychic, and mental aspects. By working in an interdependent manner, we often realize that ailments are messages from the body that can be treated by exercises and by working on the emotional and mental levels. I do my best to create a reassuring environment, so our sessions are based on trust and a feeling of well-being. This is necessary for putting clients at ease, so they can relax and find an emotional connection. That is how you will find the source of your problems, too. I suggest you use the same approach to get optimal results during your individual practice.

Seventeen years ago, at the beginning of my practice in Geneva, I was surprised to discover the extent to which the human being functions as a whole, which made me realize that that physical re-education is not enough. It is good to go beyond that to understand why pain is present. If the problem is not solved, it pops up somewhere else, sometimes with chronic tension and added intensity.

Again, this morning, I had a touching experience. At 8 am, my first client, coming because of tingling sensations in her arms and pain in her neck, told me she knew why she had those ailments. After extensive investigation, her doctor confirmed it was not a disc hernia or arthrosis; in fact, he did not find any mechanical explanation. She also shared with me that her 12-year-old daughter suffered from anorexia and that my client felt powerless. Her arms, representing her ability to move things around, were painful, and she could barely move them. When her daughter had started taking anti-anxiety medication two weeks before, she had started eating a little more, and the pain in my client's arms lessened. She told me she knew perfectly well that it was because she was relieved by the medication's effect on her daughter; now, her presence and good intentions are useful. She can now support her child.

This was the first time she had talked to someone about this problem, and the tension in her neck was dissipating slowly because she could finally express her pain in words. Of course, my program of positions, reinforcement, and flexibility had contributed to that. The key was that, through those exercises, my client was more in tune with her body. A trusting relationship had been created, and she felt safe, which allowed her to express her suffering.

Starting with Yin Yoga poses has been proven. This slow, profound practice, which is especially accessible to everyone, requires letting go, which promotes an interior state of well-being. At the beginning, the hardest part is to remain still and hold those positions for a long time. Being able to do that is a learning process about letting go and the connection with breathing so the muscles, ligaments, tendons, and fasciae can relax. If you listen to yourself, breathing has a lot of power. Breathing is living. But it is quite usual not to be conscious of your breathing. I would go even further—that it is completely ignored. I have had consultations for states of chronic fatigue, the cause of which was often superficial breathing, which consequently reduced vital energy from a lack of oxygen.

Integrating breathing exercises, *pranayamas* (see Chapter 9 about anxiety) allows you to notice your breathing and re-discover your vitality. That state precedes meditation and creative visualization because *pranayamas* invite you into an introspective state, allowing a deep calm to settle in.

Add to that the physical benefits of Yin Yoga, like the recovery of your flexibility or the elimination of arthrosis pain and a sedentary lifestyle (with age, collagen levels, and flexibility decrease), and you will not be tempted to forgo this practice.

It was also dear to my heart to integrate therapeutic visualization into my life. I did that at 15 and I continue to see its effectiveness and importance every day. I am convinced that connecting with your deep emotions brings you a comprehension of your own being beyond anything you could have experienced before.

Understanding your functioning and what you need to be happy are the first steps of this technique. Taking them brings you to understand what is upsetting you, and then you can meditate on how to face your problems. Recognizing your ailments, understanding the message your body is trying to transmit to you, and using Yin Yoga poses can help you on your self-healing path.

I hope you will find inspiration in a Yin Yoga practice.

What is Yin Yoga?

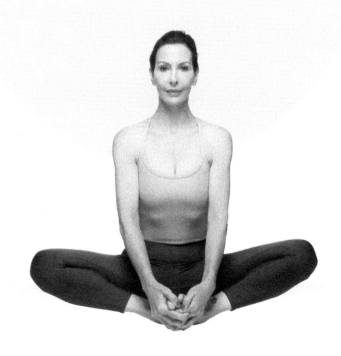

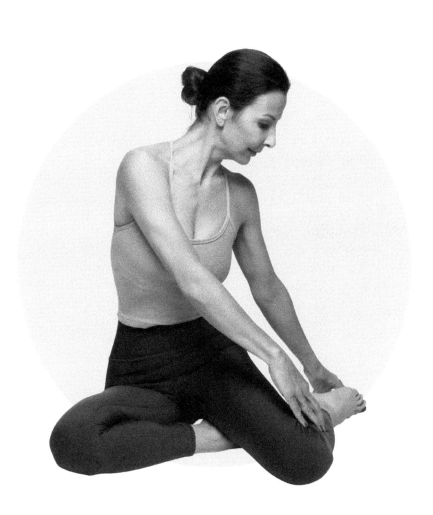

Yin Yoga is a rather passive form of yoga in which you maintain the poses for many minutes to allow you deeper into the practice. That way, you gain more flexibility by working out muscles, tendons, and ligaments, and the conjunctive tissues of the fasciae, which allow you to become more flexible.

Yin yoga promotes a meditative state. The connection between mind, body, and spirit is stimulated. You learn to listen to yourself and to know yourself better. You meet and directly face your emotions. You can then talk about full consciousness; during your therapy sessions, this is essential. We integrate self-healing skills. That means that you learn to observe yourself to know yourself better. That enables you to find solutions to your life problems and, eventually, to understand which behavior to change, so things get better. Sometimes, your point of view changes with time, so you face some personal obstacles differently and find some solutions. This behavior change can create habits which help to forge your personality later. Yin Yoga is a therapeutic method accessible to everyone.

What are the benefits of this style of Yoga?

Yin Yoga improves blood circulation and anchors you in the present moment. Its calming and soothing effect, induced by slow, intense breathing, eases into a meditative state. It allows stress and anxiety to dissipate. You benefit from the relaxation of the fasciae, which reduces joint and muscular pain. Yin brings relaxation and deeper breathing.

You benefit from greater mobility and flexibility of your joints and can then move with greater ease. Indeed, the positions stretch, compress, and twist some tissues of your body, which circulates the liquid in the joint capsules, thus preventing their deterioration, and ligament atrophy. With Yin, you allow your body to benefit from deep yet soft stretching.

Yin Yoga considers the body, the mind, and the spirit. You stimulate the energy of your body, as well as your mental and emotional states.

Chakras and meridians are deeply affected by this practice. They promote the circulation of Prana and Chi, the life energy within our being.

Yin's History

The spiritual way and yoga took form in India over 5,000 years ago. Those teachings have been transmitted through time and beyond that country.

Spirituality adapts to culture and, thus, changes. What was more directed towards the spirit and breathing in Europe is more directed towards Prana in India and Chi in China.

In Taoism, it is possible to find many spiritual practices, like the principles of the eight elements of Raja Yoga from the Yoga Sutras. Living according to the Taoism philosophy and Vedic scriptures means watching your lifestyle, respecting the correct rules of ethical behavior, and practicing yoga's breathing exercises and postures to maintain internal balance. Chi and Prana can then flow freely and bring you to a harmonious, peaceful life.

TAO

Tao, defined as the path of life, finds its balance between the forces of Yin and Yang. You feel a profound balance and a state of abundance.

Taoism is one of the three pillars of the Chinese thought, along with Confucianism and Buddhism. Those concepts have played an important role in the development of Chinese thinking. Taoism can be interpreted as a lifestyle and as the capacity to adapt to constant change. Tao philosophy is documented in the famous and popular book from Lao Tzu *Tao te Ching*, composed of 81 short and deeply moving poems.

I would like to mention my favorite poem.

TAO TE CHING

Align body and soul so they sail in unison and do not get apart.

Focus on one's vital force and make it docile like the one of a newborn.

Beyond reality, scrutinize the polished mirror by the look of the soul and let yourself be sucked into the luminous darkness.

Spare the people without intervening.

Remain calm, like the woman, when the doors of existence open and close.

Keep your ignorance and see things in their light.

Give life and protect it.

Produce without appropriating.

Act expecting nothing.

Lead without dominating.

This is the path of the mysterious perfection.

You will ask what the principles of those Chinese philosophies are. They are based on the following elements, according to Confucius:

1 The Path (Tao)
2 The Vital Breath (Qi)
3 Human Virtue (Ren).

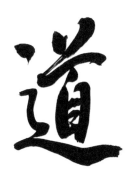

The Path: Tao

Tao is a substantial aspect of Chinese philosophy which can be translated as "The Path." Its fundamental force flows in everything within the universe and is considered the Mother of the World. Tao is the necessary matrix within the world to allow the passage of Qi and the parity between Yin and Yang.

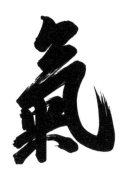

The Vital Breath, Chi, Life Energy: Qi

This symbol comes from Chinese and Japanese cultures (Ki). Its translation is not apparent but refers to a fluid that is not perceivable, often cataloged as air, creating the universe. It is an esoteric notion that connects living beings and things throughout the planet.

Within Taoism, a spiritual approach defines Chi as a breath circulating throughout the universe, simultaneously the source of life and what perpetuates it.

I find it very similar to Prana, a Sanskrit term from yoga's philosophical writings. It is often seen, especially in Hinduism, the Upanishads, and the Yoga Sutra. Prana is the breath, the vital energy that is omnipresent. The Upanishads mainly speak of Atman, "the individual," and Brahman, "the universe." One is part of the other reciprocally. Prana is present within both elements. Like Chi, it is not only the air but the universal energy everywhere. There is Prana and Chi everywhere, sometimes a bit less, sometimes a bit more, in a state of permanent flux.

Human Virtue (Ren)

The moral ideal presented by Confucius is that of the good man, literally the "noble man," which he opposes to the "man of little." With Confucius, this "nobility" takes a moral meaning. Contrary to the "man of little" who only sees his profit, the good man practices the perfect virtue (Ren) or, at least, aspires to it, as far as sacrificing his life if needed. This perfect virtue is often called "human sense," because of its similarity with the word human and its graphic character, which seems to represent the relation between two human beings.

Back then, even Confucius thought he was far away from the perfect virtue. However, this virtue is not an inaccessible goal. He who ardently desires it already possesses it within himself. Although he often spoke about that virtue, Confucius rarely defined it. However, he said that the perfect virtue is to love others. In this love, we begin by establishing ourselves. We can then draw on ourselves, allowing others to improve themselves. This virtue cannot be separated from the righteousness of the heart and of leniency that the master defines as not doing to others what you would not want them to do to you. The perfect virtue also includes the concretization of virtues relevant to the social context. Filial piety towards parents and specific loyalties towards the sovereign stem from this, and towards friends. These have become fundamental concepts of Chinese morality.

The Yin and Yang Principle

In Chinese philosophy, including Taoism, Yin and Yang represent two opposite energies, the masculine and the feminine, the active and the calm. They are simultaneous, contrary, interconnected, and complementary.

Yin	Yang
Dark	Luminous
Passive	Active
Night	Day
Equal	Unequal
Water	Fire
Empty	Empty

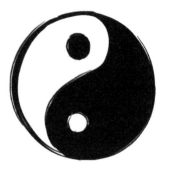

Those two energies pass through the meridians and contribute to the optimal organization of the organs. For our body, spirit, and soul to function in a balanced and harmonious way, both Yin and Yang aspects must be equally represented and developed. Without that, health problems arise, like an alarm reminding us to act and keep listening to ourselves.

We clearly live in a society oriented towards the Yang. We need to be active and dynamic, and to constantly perform. This lifestyle can lead to burnout and unhealthy escape mechanisms. To compensate and maintain the pace imposed by the environment, and often by ourselves, we continue to pull on the rope until our body imposes a rest period on us.

It is, of course, equally possible to be too much in the Yin, the passive, which can lead to depressive states as well as emotional and material dependence. Do you always need to have someone to help you finish your projects and stand? You need more dynamism (Yang) and rational action to create a healthy balance and find your life's vitality. Homeostasis depends on the principle of Yin and Yang. Any imbalance can deplete your internal and external resources, weaken your resilience, and lead you to exhaustion.

Yin Yoga represents an extraordinary way to integrate more calm, passive energy into your life. To create personal balance and harmony, the combined practice of Yin and Yang is perfect. Why not start with a more dynamic series of Yang postures, then continue with calm and rejuvenating Yin postures?

In my opinion, it is essential to analyze where you are on your personal path, then evaluate which of those two aspects needs to be developed further. The goal is always to live in the daylight and to rest at night.

The Anatomy and Physiology of the Human Body

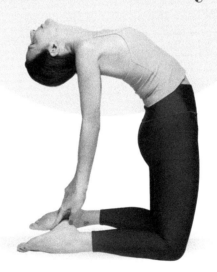

Your body comprises bones, muscles, ligaments, tendons, and fasciae. In Yin Yoga practice, the fasciae are critical.

The skeletal system

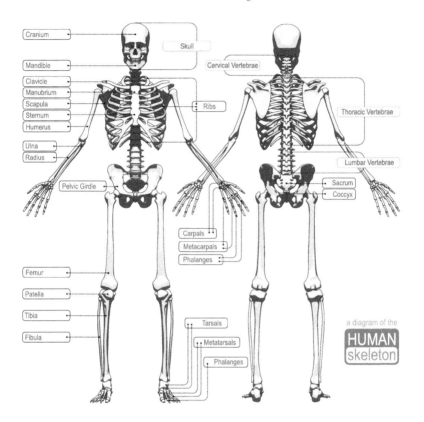

Cranium

Skull

Mandible

Cervical Vertebrae

Clavicle

Manubrium

Scapula

Ribs

Sternum

Humerus

Thoracic Vertebrae

Ulna

Radius

Lumbar Vertebrae

Pelvic Girdle

Sacrum

Coccyx

Carpals

Metacarpals

Phalanges

Femur

Patella

Tibia

Tarsals

Fibula

Metatarsals

Phalanges

a diagram of the

HUMAN skeleton

The basis of the skeletal system is the spine, made of bone components (vertebrae) and inter-vertebral discs acting as shock absorbers between adjacent vertebrae. The spine ensures cohesion and mobility. You have many types of vertebrae: seven cervical, 12 dorsal, five lumbar, a sacrum composed of five welded vertebrae, and finally, a coccyx at the bottom of the spine, four atrophied, welded vertebrae.

The spine is not only significant physically; it is also fundamental on the energetic level. Kundalini, vital energy, flows all along it, running up as two energy canals, the nadis. The two nadis (ida and pingala) go up and cross each other along the sushumna, the spine, to create the chakras. Healthy and mobile vertebrae are the sign of a life full of energy and creative force.

Conjunctive Tissue

All the organs of a body are organized around conjunctive tissue, which comprises fibers and is essential to the good functioning of the body. Conjunctive tissues act as support, protect other tissues, and look after functional tissues by supplying nutrient and disposing of waste.

There are three kinds of conjunctive tissue:

- Tissue which supports the various structures of the organs, veins, bones, muscles, etc.
- Connective tissue between the articular and peri-articular structures – the joints. This is very rich in collagen, the substance that hold bones, tendons, skin and blood vessels together.
- Conjunctive tissue in bone tissue.

This tissue is present everywhere in the body in different forms and for different functions. Yin Yoga strengthens it and makes it flexible.

Yin Yoga has more effect on the conjunctive tissues of:

- The ligaments.
- The tendons.
- Articulations.
- Fasciae.

Tendons

Tendons connect muscles and bones. They are strong and flexible, so they can maintain a certain pressure. They have sensors to alert us in the case of excessive stretching. Some cells flag to the nervous systems to relax the muscle connected to the bone quickly. The elastic limit of a tendon is only about 4%. If you try to stretch a tendon beyond that, you risk permanent damage. This explains why it is essential to enter the Yin Yoga postures slowly and not go too far. Stop when you feel a stretch is too intense and be patient. With time, tendons, ligaments, fasciae, and muscles will become more flexible and allow you to go further with no effort.

Achilles Tendon

calf muscle

Achilles tendon

heel

Ligaments

A ligament is a short band of very strong conjunctive fibrous tissue that connects one bone to another within an articulation. They look like tendons but are much darker.

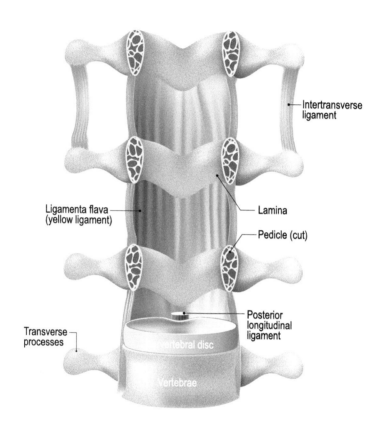

Intertransverse ligament

Ligamenta flava (yellow ligament)

Lamina

Pedicle (cut)

Transverse processes

Posterior longitudinal ligament

Vertebral disc

Vertebrae

Ligaments are made of collagen, which explains their mechanical strength and stability. When elastic fibers grow old, they mineralize and cross each other, which is responsible for the loss of flexibility.

Articulations (joints)

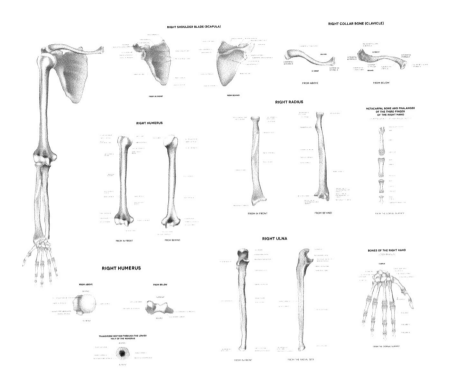

An articulation is a junction zone between two bone endings.
Bones of the Upper Extremities

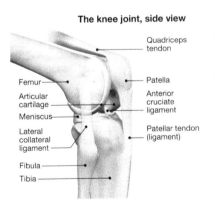

The knee joint, side view

Quadriceps tendon

Femur

Patella

Articular cartilage

Anterior cruciate ligament

Meniscus

Lateral collateral ligament

Patellar tendon (ligament)

Fibula

Tibia

A joint's mobility depends on its constitution, its shape and the nature of the surrounding elements. Joints are moved by the skeletal muscles. Their other function is to support the body.

The fluid in the joint capsules deteriorates when you are not moving enough. This is clearly a problem with our modern sedentary society. I thus strongly recommend that you integrate the practice of yoga into your daily life to increase your quality of life. It is the only discipline considering the body, the mind, and the soul while respecting their connection and interdependency.

Yoga allows you to confer flexibility and strength on your muscles simultaneously. It is a perfect combination that allows aging with minimal loss of agility and flexibility.

Collagen – the body's 'glue'

Tendons and ligaments are made of collagen, a protein that provides mechanical resistance to tissues when stretching. Collagen is the most influential protein in the human body as it is a major component of the conjunctive tissues, including the tendons, ligaments, skin, and muscles.

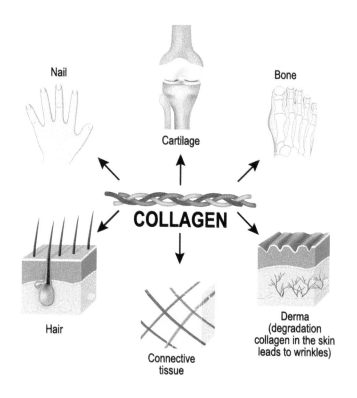

It is also found in bones, blood vessels, and the digestive system. It contributes to the strength and elasticity of our tissues. In simple terms, it is the "glue" helping to keep our bodies together.

Age-related collagen reduction

Collagen production in our body slows down naturally with age. We can notice this degenerative process by the signs of aging, wrinkles, sagging skin, and joint pain. However, Yin Yoga maintains the body's flexibility. That's one more reason to practice it!

Fasciae – the vital connective tissue

Fasciae have become a trendy theme! They had been ignored for a long time, but nowadays everyone is talking about them and their importance. Scientific research is in progress, and knowledge keeps growing.

We now know that fasciae are conjunctive tissues which are very rich in the collagen fibers responsible for flexibility and potential pain. It's thanks to them that you can stand up. Indeed, they are connected to form a global conjunctive tissue, maintaining the body and connecting each of its parts.

The name "fascia" comes from Latin and means strip. You can imagine fasciae as like the white tissue that covers the interior of an orange. It is flexible, elastic tissue enveloping muscles, ligaments, tendons, bones, and organs to form something like a bag around them.

When you move and stretch your articulations enough, fasciae are flexible and fluid. The water and hyaluronic acid in fasciae play a decisive role in their flexibility and functionality. A lack of physical activity and stretching causes stiffening and water loss, directly affecting flexibility and mobility, and causing pain.

The fasciae represent a large part of the human body, but they do not appear on anatomy illustrations, although they are visible to the naked eye and are very important.

Interestingly, it has been scientifically proven that some hormonal biochemical messages, especially from emotional stress, can contract fasciae independently from a muscular or nervous stimulus.

There are different types of fasciae:

- Superficial fasciae, also called subcutaneous tissues, are a deep layer of the skin.

- Deep fasciae, harder and less flexible, are separate superficial muscles from the subcutaneous tissue.

- Internal fasciae fill space between the organs.

- Visceral fasciae take care of the suspension and framing of the internal organs.

Fasciae have a fluid constitution and are easily displaced. What is fascinating is that they can react independently of what they wrap. A fascia wrapping a muscle can contract independently of the muscle because it has more nerve endings. Consequently, it is possible for you to feel pain originating from some fasciae and not the muscles they wrap around. In such a case, giving flexibility to your fasciae will eliminate the pain. Muscular massages will have only a short-term effect, because the source of the ailment is not the muscle. The explanation is simply that the fasciae are sensory organs, while muscles are not, and as such, they transmit sensory information to the central nervous system.

Other sensory organs include the eyes, the ears, the tongue, and the skin. The cells and tissues of those organs, including the fasciae, receive messages and translate them to signals that can be understood and used by the nervous system.

Dr. Robert Schleip, researcher at the Ulm University (Germany) and fasciae specialist, has shown that stretching joints to the maximum in all directions gives and maintains flexibility to fasciae, so you can regain all lost flexibility and lose pain.

To practice Yin Yoga and its flexibility exercises correctly, you need to know your body and which of the three flexibility types you have:

- Hypermobility.
- the flexibility of the Viking.
- the crossover, named by its inventor, the Czech Dr. Vladimir Janda, (1928–2002).

Your flexibility depends on:

- genetic factors. Women are generally more flexible than men.
- heredity. Within the same family, you can often see identical postural types, similar morphology, strength, and flexibility, and this has been scientifically proven.

Hypermobility

When flexibility is dominant in relation to strength, you can often see the hypermobility of joints.

I always use a plumb line to analyze posture. It is a vertical line that, in the case of a perfect posture, goes from the ear to the shoulder, the femur's head, the knee, and the heel. When the knees are behind that line, they are hyperlaxed or hypermobile.

Another example is elbows. When you extend your arm, if the elbow joint is deviated laterally and not aligned with the head of the humerus and the wrist, it is hyperlaxed.

Any hyperlaxed joint requires more fascial tone to better

support and protect it. Regarding your Yin Yoga practice, that translates to not holding a pose to your flexibility's limit. On the contrary, you look for a pose where you must hold yourself back, to give tone to your fasciae. This will give you better joint support.

Harmony between strength and flexibility, Yin and Yang, brings a physical and psychic balance, giving you the balance necessary to live peacefully without pain.

The flexibility of the Viking

The Viking Disease, also called Dupuytren's contracture, is related to palmar fasciae that can lead to a progressive flexion of one or more fingers. The individual suffering from this pathology is subject to lost mobility of those fingers. For a while now, the increased flexibility of fasciae has been proven. It has also been shown that working on that conjunctive tissue can help regain finger mobility.

If genetically, you have little flexibility, it is imperative to promote the flexibility of the fasciae during the practice of Yin Yoga. That means finding poses that allow you to relax, soften your fasciae, and keep the pose for at least three minutes, with the help of accessories (cushion, blanket, blocks, belt, etc.), if necessary.

The Crossover type

Dr. Janda is the creator of the definition of the lower crossed syndrome, or "crossover," referring to a muscular imbalance and dysfunction in the hip region. This imbalance largely comes from prolonged sitting, which is omnipresent in our lifestyle involving office work, driving cars, eating at restaurants, etc.

This posture places the hip flexor muscles, mainly the psoas and iliac muscles, in a shortened position for a long time.

Characteristics of **the lower-crossed syndrome** are a weakening of the abdominal muscles and the *gluteus maximus*, as well as atrophy of the *quadrature lumborum* muscle. The body adapts to function and rebalances the system so it can perform, but you will suffer from the atrophy's consequences: tension and back pain settle chronically within your life, and posture changes require a correction to not worsen.

The **upper-crossed syndrome** causes muscular dysfunction in the upper part of the body. As with the lower crossed syndrome, it results from our lifestyle. People suffering from this syndrome have a head-forward posture, cervical hyperlordosis, dorsal hyperkyphosis, and elevation and protraction of the shoulders. The weakened muscles are the rhomboids and the lower trapezius, while the tensed muscles are the large and small pectorals and the upper trapezius.

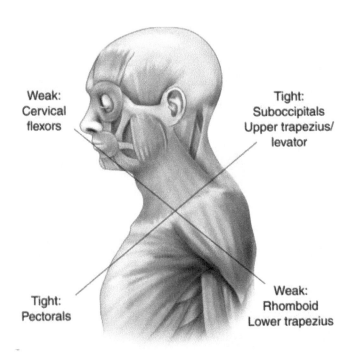

Weak:
Cervical
flexors

Tight:
Suboccipitals
Upper trapezius/
levator

Tight:
Pectorals

Weak:
Rhomboid
Lower trapezius

Dr. Janda has published 16 books and was one of the first to have studied medicine and physiotherapy. He has devoted a large part of his life to research to rebalancing the imbalances[1] of the locomotor system. He judges it is essential to determine which muscles and joints are flexible and strong, to balance the agonist and the antagonist (the muscle that creates the movement and the one that stabilizes it), and the whole body. You need to identify which muscles are flexible and which ones are rigid, and work accordingly.

For your practice of Yin Yoga, that means that hyperlaxed joints must be toned and strengthened by avoiding going to the limit of your capacity. Rigid joints will gain deep flexibility and reach physical harmony.

Fascia-Related Pain

As mentioned, a sedentary lifestyle, a lack of movement, and poor posture knot the fasciae because of a lack of lubrication. Pain appears, and you lose flexibility. To better explain the difference between muscular and fascial pain, I refer to the study carried out by Heidelberg University. A painful substance was injected into the quadrature lumborum muscle and into the fasciae of the same area. The muscular discomfort was easy to determine, and it was possible to point at it with a finger. For the fasciae, the region was much larger, about the size of the palm. It was scientifically proven that 10% to 15% of back pain is because of vertebrae and that the rest, 80% to 85%, is more related to the fasciae.

The fasciae take part in your proprioception. The word "proprio" is taken from the Latin proprius (own) and "[re]ception" (deep sensibility). It designates our perception, conscious or not, of the position of the different parts of our body, knowing where

---

1. Muscular imbalances are at the root of locomotor system problems.

the limbs of the body are and being aware of their movement.

The fasciae are passive and react to our senses and emotions. They can contract and influence our muscular dynamic. If you are stressed or tense, this will affect them, and they will lose flexibility. Cortisol, the stress hormone being transmitted through this conjunctive tissue, is responsible for that.

That also goes the other way. If you are happy and joyful, your posture is open; your back is well stretched, and you produce hormones like serotonin, which gives you a feeling of well-being. The fasciae can work perfectly, and your joints are then soft and flexible.

I think a good posture is the basis of a balanced body and mind.

I often hear my clients complain about pain in their hips and shoulders. We often discover that they carry the weight of the world on their shoulders. Working on the relaxation of the fasciae is a proven therapeutic approach. As for hip pain, we need to understand that the hips are considered the "trashcan" of emotions. They have a lot of nerve endings, and since the *iliopsoas* is the only muscle connecting the top and the bottom of the body, toxins easily accumulate there. The proximity of the digestive system and the eliminating organs also promote this accumulation.

I can give you two tips to solve those tensions:

- a physical approach: stretch out the iliopsoas, which you can achieve by practicing the Dragon, for example.

- an emotional approach: live your emotions fully and take the time to be present in the moment. Digest your emotions. Ignoring or avoiding them will inevitably lead to physical or psychological blockages.

That is why Yin Yoga seems to be a form of very efficient therapy; you are listening to your body and your mind.

Something else that can be prevented with this form of therapy is the loss of flexibility resulting from age and a sedentary lifestyle. The best way to prevent it is to be active and to ensure your posture is optimal. If you have bad posture (through heredity, linked to your mood or some pain) and do not correct it for a while, fasciae lose the ability to straighten you.

It's a good idea to see your body as a whole and not isolate the tender parts. You can feel those fascial knots as hardness in some places under the skin. Almost all chronic pains are caused by fasciae that have lost their elasticity. This problem can be treated by massage therapists, acupuncturists, or yoga therapists.

Ideally, it is useful to combine Yin and Yang practices. But what does that mean ? A Yang sport is fast and strengthens your muscles with repetitive movements and impacts that have to be absorbed by your joints. A Yin practice works softly on the fasciae. You need to take the time to stay in your postures and listen to yourself. To strengthen muscles, improve cardio, relax the fasciae and get the most benefit, combine both!

Skeletal Muscle

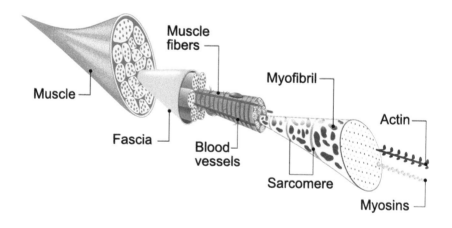

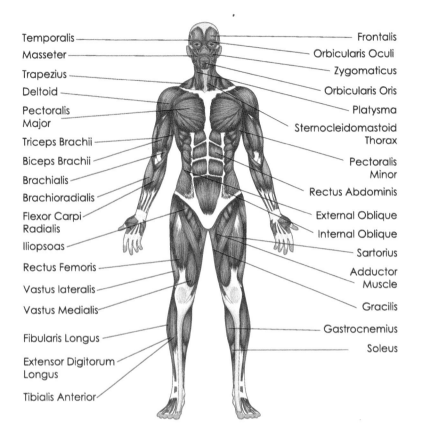

Temporalis
Masseter
Trapezius
Deltoid
Pectoralis Major
Triceps Brachii
Biceps Brachii
Brachialis
Brachioradialis
Flexor Carpi Radialis
Iliopsoas
Rectus Femoris
Vastus lateralis
Vastus Medialis
Fibularis Longus
Extensor Digitorum Longus
Tibialis Anterior

Frontalis
Orbicularis Oculi
Zygomaticus
Orbicularis Oris
Platysma
Sternocleidomastoid
Thorax
Pectoralis Minor
Rectus Abdominis
External Oblique
Internal Oblique
Sartorius
Adductor Muscle
Gracilis
Gastrocnemius
Soleus

Muscular tissues

The human body has:

- smooth cardiac muscular tissue.
- skeletal muscular tissue.

Smooth cardiac muscles are under the control of the parasympathetic autonomic nervous system and facilitate our physical functions, such as digestion and heartbeat. On the other hand, skeletal muscles are used to move our body in space and move the bones, as their name implies. There are over 600 muscles in your body, representing about 40% of your body mass.

Skeletal muscles are tied to a bone or a joint. When the insertion and origin points of the muscle get closer, we call it a concentric contraction. Imagine, for example, that the elbow joint bends, muscles then pull on the radius and ulna, and on the bones of the forearm. The insertion and origin points of the biceps get closer, which creates a concentric contraction. When you extend the arm, those two points get farther apart, and it is called an eccentric contraction because the muscle extends.

Most of the skeletal muscles work that way. There are only a few muscles that simply change volume, the ones that contract isometrically, meaning by changing volume, but not length: the multifidus, the pelvic floor, and the transverse and the abdominal diaphragm.

In Yin Yoga, we mostly use the skeletal muscles.

Stabilizing muscles

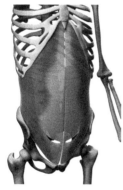

Stabilizing muscles work with slow muscular fibers (pelvic floor, *transversus abdominis* muscle, diaphragm, and *multifidus*). Their ability to maintain and support your organs and posture is infinite, because they activate only 20% of their maximum strength. You can thus maintain your back straight all day long.

Transverse abdomen muscle - *transversus abdominis*

The transversus abdominis muscle is the deepest and most significant in the abdominal zone. It acts as a stabilizer and intervenes to maintain a good posture. Its other function is to protect the internal organs. Because it is isometric and deep, making it invisible, sadly, this muscle is little known. Contrary to a mobilizing muscle like the biceps, which can contract in a concentric or eccentric manner, an isometric muscle

cannot change length. Especially with its toning, there will be
a refinement of your silhouette. Moreover, your back pain will
disappear.

The pelvic floor

The pelvic floor is also a stabilizing muscle. It is the source of
the first chakra, *Muladhara*, and a stabilizer of the chest. With
the *transversus* and the *multifidus*, it ensures the support of the
organs and good posture. A weakening of this muscle causes
tension, even pain, in the back and can lead to incontinence and
prolapse.

From the illustration you can see that your pelvis comprises:

- iliac crests
- pubic symphysis
- seat bones
- coccyx
- sacrum
- sacroiliac joint.

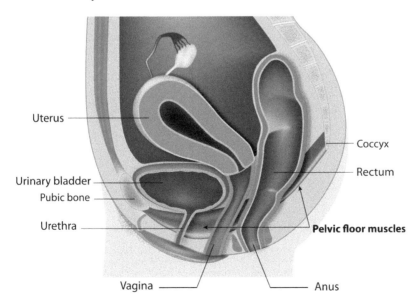

Uterus

Coccyx

Rectum

Urinary bladder

Pubic bone

Urethra

Pelvic floor muscles

Vagina

Anus

It is possible to distinguish three muscular layers. The deepest are the *levator ani* muscle and the *ischio-coccygeal* muscle.

On the second level, there are the deep *transversus*, the sphincter and urethra.

Finally, on the surface, there are: the anus, superficial *transversus* muscles, *bulbo* and *ischiocavernosus*, which are the builders of the vulva in women.

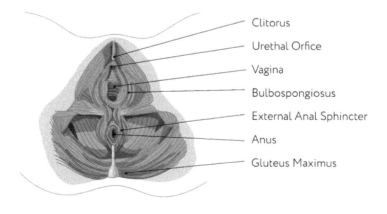

Clitorus

Urethal Orfice

Vagina

Bulbospongiosus

External Anal Sphincter

Anus

Gluteus Maximus

Vulva

The masculine and feminine pelvic floors are different in two respects. The first is the size; the masculine pelvic floor is narrower, while the feminine is wider to allow for reproduction. In addition, the female includes the vulva and the anus, separated by a skin area. That fibrous zone is precisely what supports the uterus and vagina. Female prolapse is the direct consequence of the destruction of this part, just like incontinence, because organ drop increases intra-abdominal pressure. Overweight, bad posture and repetitive impacts can also cause prolapse. Men can also suffer from a weak pelvic floor, which causes lower back pain.

The multifidus - Multifidus Spinae, Multifidi

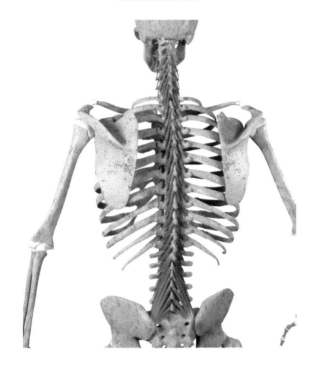

The *multifidus* is a slow fiber muscle able to contract only in an isometry. It starts around the axis (vertebra #2) and stretches vertically along the entire spine down to the sacrum. It is divided into sections: the cervical multifidus, dorsal multifidus, and lumbar multifidus. More precisely, it begins at the C4 vertebra and is tied to the sacrum.

The resulting stiffness allows each vertebra to function more efficiently and reduces the degeneration of joint structures caused by friction during daily movements. The multifidus greatly contributes to the local stability of the spine, along with transverse abdominal muscle, among others.

This muscle is a key element in back re-education and the maintenance of good posture. Often ignored, it suffers the same fate as the transversus and the pelvic floor and passes under the radar because it is not directly visible, and its strengthening is done through a more subtle approach. Since it comprises slow muscle fibers and cannot move bones, we need to realize that strengthening a stabilization muscle does not provide us with the same sensations of burning and fatigue as the strengthening of a mobilization muscle. You will feel lifted and toned but not exhausted. Toning it relieves back pains, thanks to better spine segment stabilization.

The benefits of strengthening the multifidus are multiple:

- an improvement of your posture, by stretching your back.
- a relief of dorsal tension, including lumbago.
- a better central stabilization of your vertebrae, and provision of the necessary anchorage to support your back and the proper posture of the body.

How to strengthen it? All Yin Yoga positions are effective if you keep in mind creating a maximum distance between the lumbar and cervical vertebrae. If you want to go further, know that the unbalanced exercises and postures have been proven, so you can use unstable surfaces for effective reinforcement.

The exercise below not only reinforces the *multifidus* but also removes intra-abdominal pressure from the pelvic floor and tones the transverse. If you do not have accessories at your disposal, place yourself on all fours and simply lift one leg along with the opposite arm. Maintain this position for three breaths. Make sure the shoulder girdle and hips remain aligned. Then, change sides. That is simple and efficient. You can also practice Yin Yoga's cat pose to harmonize the energies within your body and relax your back.

Mobilizing Muscles

The other skeletal muscles are the mobilizing muscles that

move joints by applying eccentric or concentric contraction principles. You can perform abductions, adductions, flexions, extensions, elevations, descents, and back and front shoulder thrusts.

Flexion and extension

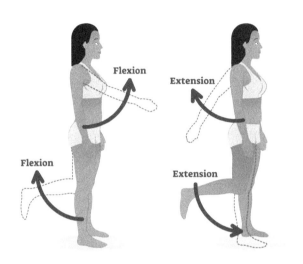

Types of Body Movement

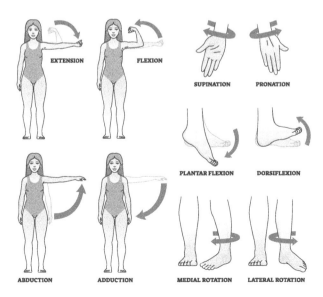

The Iliopsoas—Pelvis

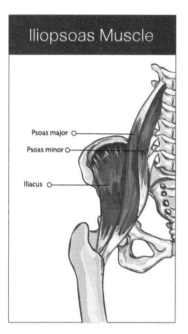

Iliopsoas Muscle

Psoas major

Psoas minor

Iliacus

One of the critical mobilization muscles is the *iliopsoas*, the only muscle connecting the body's top and bottom. It is in fact made up of three different muscles: the *psoas major*, the *psoas minor* (which today has lost its importance as some people no longer have it), and the iliac muscle. The major and minor *psoas* usually work in tandem with the lumbar muscles *(quadratus lumborum)*.

The major *psoas* connects the femur and the pelvis (iliac crest), and thus, the top and bottom of the body. The minor *psoas* connects the pelvis (iliac crest) and the spine and does not contribute much to the body's movement. The iliac muscle is just added to the *psoas*. This is the deepest and strongest hip flexor. It starts from the femur and goes towards the iliac bone.

The primary function of the *iliopsoas* is the flexion of the hips. It also helps the *quadratus lumborum* muscle to stabilize the spine. These muscles flex the torso beyond 30° and also contribute to the abduction and internal rotation of the femur.

The *psoas major* determines the position of the pelvis. It is inserted from T12 (thoracic vertebra 12) to L4 and L5 (lumbar vertebrae 4 and 5), and passes inside the iliac crest to connect to the great trochanter. If it is too short, it increases the camber, and it is then necessary to stretch it to relieve the back. You can achieve that by practicing Yin's posture of the Pigeon.

Your muscles can stretch 50% to 60% compared to their resting length. As you grow older or after injury, you lose flexibility and movement amplitude. Consequently, your muscles atrophy. The number of nerve cells reduces; muscles change their constitution by turning into fat tissue, called collagen, which resists stretching. However, you can slow and reverse this process by practicing Yin Yoga regularly.

Other physical activities strengthen muscles, indeed, but concentric work, which is often explosive, does not stretch them at all. On the contrary, it gives them rigidity. Only by practicing yoga can you unite mind, spirit, and soul while you reinforce and stretch your body.

Different Postural Types and Back Pathologies

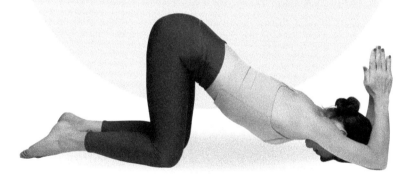

This chapter discusses the different postural types and back pathologies and their emotional origins. It is crucial to define the human being as a body-mind-soul unit, especially when it concerns back pain.

The spine is the rope of our back. It represents strength and stability.

How do you go about your life? Hunched, or straight and proud? Everything is linked! What I am saying is illustrated by the popular expression "I carry the world on my shoulders." I stopped counting the number of clients suffering from chronic pain without a medical diagnosis. This is not because they have not consulted. On the contrary, it is stress and anxiety that trigger your alarm. Listen to your symptoms, search to understand the underlying message and treat yourself correctly.

Often, this pain comes up during stressful periods of your life. Take the time to analyze them. The reason this pain appears is often deeper than you think. Do not forget that before the appearance of intense pain, you have probably ignored something. In a self-healing process, it is suggested that you note every detail (situations, emotions, etc.) preceding the acute pain to understand and solve your problem.

The Spine

A spine has two curves (lordoses), the cervical and lumbar lordoses. The spine's role is to support and protect the spinal cord. In total, it includes 33 vertebrae, stacked vertically, each one on top of another; seven cervical vertebrae, 12 dorsal vertebrae, five lumbar vertebrae, vertebrae welded together forming the coccyx, and another group of welded vertebrae forming the sacrum.

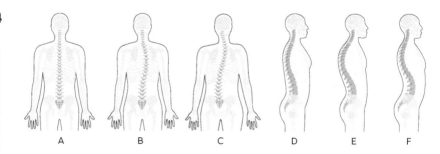

A: Normal spine B. Thoracic scoliosis C: Combined scoliosis
D: Normal spine E: Kyphosis F: Lordosis

Scoliosis

A scoliosis is a spinal deviation. In most cases, it deviates towards the right at the height of the dorsal vertebrae. We distinguish between idiopathic and secondary scolioses. The origin of idiopathic scoliosis is unknown. It essentially appears during childhood and adolescence. My experience shows a hereditary factor, since several members of the same family can develop it. Idiopathic scolioses represent 70% to 80% of all scolioses.

A secondary scoliosis is caused by congenital malformation, neuromuscular disease or even bone disease. One leg being longer than the other can also be responsible for an asymmetry of the hips, which can lead to scoliosis. Bad posture, sports or frequently carrying a bag on the same side are obviously not related to the origin of this type of scoliosis.

When I do a postural analysis at the beginning of our session, I ask my clients to bend forward. When there is scoliosis, a bump on the side of the back is visible, a "gibbosity."

There are many symptoms of scoliosis, including tension and pain around the scapulas and sometimes, low back pain can be observed when the deviation happens at the level of the lumbar vertebrae.

Symptoms of scoliosis:

- Bad posture
- Frequent back pain
- Shallow breathing
- Fatigue from a hunched torso
- Unfavorable aesthetic appearance
- Reduction in height from the spinal deformation

How to treat this problem

To correct a scoliosis, and get rid of the tension in the middle of your back, I recommend you practice some back-twisting and stretching postures:

1. **Matsendrasana—the seated twist pose**
2. **Marjarasana—the cat pose to relax the spine**
3. **Jathara Parivartanasana—the reclining twist pose**
4. **Salabhasana—the grasshopper pose to stretch and muscle the back.**

The emotional symbolism of a scoliosis

Scoliosis often appears during childhood and adolescence. Behind that fact, something hides in some people sometimes: a profound refusal to grow up. The deviation of the spine slows down, even stops, growth. Surrounding adults and other people in charge can trigger the desire to remain a child. I have met teenagers suffering from scoliosis who gained up to 4 cm (1.5 in) after being operated on. But we need to know that surgery is rare and that it is possible to notice a significant correction of the spine by practicing the exercises below. I suggest you analyze this refusal to grow and the potential causes of that "curved" position. You need to stay straight in terms of posture but also in terms of character. To reinforce your ability to self-heal, be aware of your value and trust yourself. Do not put yourself down; you are capable.

Kyphosis

A kyphosis is a back deformation caused by the excessive curvature of the spine between the 1st and 12th vertebra. When associated with scoliosis, it is a kyphoscoliosis.

There are three types of kyphosis:

- postural kyphosis.
- Scheuermann's disease.
- kyphosis linked to age and osteoporosis.

Postural kyphosis simply designates a bad posture because of weak muscles in the trapezius and rhomboids (upper and middle back). To improve it, all you need to do is to practice stretching exercises for the pectorals and strengthening exercises for the back.

Scheuermann's disease is caused by a growth anomaly of the dorsal vertebrae. It can only be diagnosed through radiography. Back stiffness and pain are linked to it, especially after spending some time seated.

Kyphosis linked to age and osteoporosis has the same consequences as the others but a different source. Up to the age of 20, your osteoblasts build more bone mass than your osteoclasts destroy. Between the ages of 20 and 30, this ratio is about the same. After 30, the destruction is more relevant. You can appreciate this by imagining it this way: Up to 20 years old, you deposit money in an account; between 20 and 30, you deposit the same amount you withdraw; after age 30, you withdraw more than you deposit. The balance you have left depends then on the initial deposits (hereditary factor, sports activity, weight, etc.).

After many years, you might notice osteopenia (low bone mass), which is not cataloged as a pathology, but it may develop into osteoporosis, a significant reduction of the bone mass responsible for some postural changes, can turn into kyphosis. Why? This mass plays a cushioning role between vertebrae, so when it decreases, the anterior and posterior planes can be impacted, leading to significant wear of the discs.

The noticeable aesthetic aspect of all types of kyphosis is a hunched back, leading to a reduced breathing capacity. Indeed, the shoulders are arched and do not allow a deep breath to be taken. One consequence is a state of chronic fatigue from a lack of oxygen. The psychological aspect is not to be neglected: being curled forward causes depression, lack of motivation, and sometimes, frustration.

How to treat kyphosis

To open the lungs and the posture, I suggest you do:

1. *Anahatasana*—the puppy dog: the three options, one after the other, are recommended to gradually opening more and more
2. *Supta Virasana*—the reclined hero pose, lying down on the bolster, arms stretched on the sides, benefits the opening of the heart
3. *Baddha Konasana*—the butterfly: lying down on a bolster
4. *Savasana*—final relaxation, with two cushions to elevate your cervical vertebrae.

The emotional symbolism of kyphosis

The first noticeable thing with kyphosis is the weight resting on the person's shoulders. This load forces them to bend forward to stay on their feet. Their rounded back then becomes their shell, a sign of protection.

To reduce the signs of kyphosis, I suggest you write down the things that weigh on you so you can make them concrete. Then, symbolically, take them and drop them on a cloud to visualize them going away to the horizon. Make every effort to ask for help and support in carrying out all those responsibilities so you can free yourself.

Hyperlordosis

Lumbar hyperlordosis is an excessive curvature near the five lumbar vertebrae of the lower back. It can be hereditary, the consequence of weakened abdominals, or of atrophy of the hip flexors.

Put yourself into an artificial hyperlordosis. You will feel a pinch in the lumbar region and the relaxation of your muscles at the back of your legs, your glutes, and the center of your body. Additionally, the pelvic floor is weakened, even if this is hard to feel.

This postural type is very common, since we spend too much time sitting down. Hip flexors that determine the position of your pelvis atrophy and cause an anteversion (hyperlordosis). Like all postural types, this is degenerative if you do not do corrective exercises. Moreover, there is a significant risk of the descent of organs and incontinence because the anteversion of the pelvis increases intra-abdominal pressure. The bladder, in the bottom right of your pelvic floor, suffers from that weight. The phenomenon is accentuated by a lack of abdominal support.

It is good to muscle up your abdominals, the backs of your legs, and your glutes and to stretch up the psoas to avoid worsening the hyperlordosis.

How to treat hyperlordosis

1. *Navasana*—the boat pose. If necessary, hold your thighs for a moment, then release your hands. Repeat this movement as often as it is necessary.
2. *Maksikanagasana*—the dragonfly pose with hands or forearms on the ground, according to your preference to stretch out the iliopsoas
3. *Salabhasana*—the grasshopper pose to muscle up the back chain
4. *Baddha Konasana*—the butterfly, on the bolster, to stabilize the back.

The emotional symbolism of a hyperlordosis

Pelvis anteversion, thus hyperlordosis, is caused by the iliopsoas being too short and stretched. This muscle is nicknamed "the muscle of the soul." Its tension hides hypersensitivity, anxiety, and even emotionality. Self-healing on the physical level is carried out by stretching the iliopsoas. If you want to work on the emotional symbolism, I suggest you write on paper what is worrying you, as well as the situations in which you are anxious or stressed.

We usually need to do this exercise many times, and regularly write down our worries because the source of the problem is deeply anchored inside us. Once integrated, you can continue by transforming stressful situations into affirmations. For example, during an exam that stresses you, thanks to this exercise, you come to deeply feel you can succeed while remaining confident and calm. Over time, you will see that the problem comes from your own doubts, and then you will change your state of mind and approach this situation positively.

Start by recognizing your hypersensitivity and accepting it. Then, write some stressful scenarios and try to change your reaction to them. Instead of putting yourself in an anxious state, take a moment to welcome your feelings. You will live them and immediately let them go.

It is useless to invest too much energy in those emotions. Try to go over them without ignoring your feelings. You will then notice your hyperlordosis stabilizing.

Hernia & protrusion

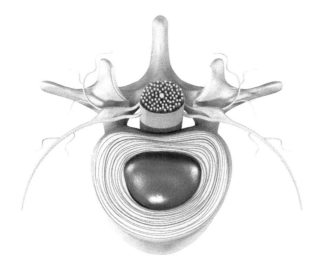

The tissues between the bones of the spine are called the intervertebral discs. They comprise a soft, gelatinous core covered by a hard shell and create a joint between each bone of the spine, allowing the bones to move. When the exterior layer of a disc tears, the soft interior substance can be pushed outside, causing a herniated disc.

Most herniated discs occur at C6 and C7 (cervical vertebrae 6 and 7), L4-L5 (lumbar vertebrae 4 and 5), or S1 (sacrum 1). The reason is simple: those are the most mobile and flexible spots, so they are more exposed and more fragile.

Cervical hernia

The first symptom of a cervical hernia is a frequent pain in the arm and the neck.

Because of my experience, I could see that many of my clients were suffering from discomfort in the shoulder area but not connecting it to their cervical vertebrae. Only after weeks of pain, and often a notable weakness in their arms, the medical diagnosis was that the pain was coming from a cervical hernia.

Lumbar hernia

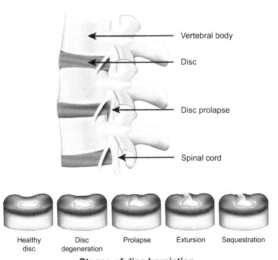

Vertebral body

Disc

Disc prolapse

Spinal cord

| Healthy disc | Disc degeneration | Prolapse | Extrusion | Sequestration |

Stages of disc herniation

The symptoms of a lumbar hernia are pain in the lower back and buttocks. If the liquid exiting the disc touches the sciatic nerve, it can irritate that nerve, leading to painful inflammation causing sciatica, that can go through the leg down to the toes.

Disc Protrusion

Each intervertebral disc has two parts, a gelatinous core of cartilage and a fibrous ring encircling it. The protrusion mechanism results from a progressive and natural deflation of the intervertebral disc, and as a result, the soft interior regularly extends around the edge of the vertebral nodes. The capacity of the liquid core in the disc's center is less effective. The liquid pressure diminishes, reducing the height of the disc while its diameter increases.

A discal hernia—often the consequence of a non-treated protrusion—is a protrusion from the normal circumference of the annulus of the intervertebral disc. If that prominence touches or compresses a nerve, it sparks pain that spreads over the length of the nerve.

It is a natural step of the spine-aging process, and the first symptoms can appear as early as 40. It can develop towards a complete and progressive disappearance of the core, starting with the lower discs, then moving up to the superior discs. People affected feel major pain in the affected region: most often in the lumbar region, less often in the cervical region, and rarely in the dorsal vertebrae.

Risk factors

- Being overweight.
- Physical jobs with repetitive movements.
- Regularly carrying heavy loads.
- Sedentary lifestyle.
- Lack of physical exercise, immobility.

How to treat disc protrusion

Since the pain is caused by the soft substance protruding from the disc, the goal is to make this substance re-enter the disc. It is simple; imagine a vertebra with its vertebral body, which is harder and provides more stability. It is thus more mobile towards the anterior and lateral zones. Because they are less protected, these sites are exactly where the substance protrudes. It is scientifically proven that this substance can retract if you do the correct movements and exercises—dorsal extensions.

Maybe you are wondering what dorsal extensions are. They are movements in which the body leans back.

I often notice that after a hernia and a protrusion, my clients suffer from a physical or psychic trauma. Practicing those intense positions can lead to tension. I suggest you begin by stretching exercises for the back to regain confidence in yourself and your body.

1. *Baddha Konasana*—the butterfly, seated with a straight back.
2. *Supta Baddha Konasana*—the relined butterfly, with or without a bolster.
3. *Paschimottanasana*—the caterpillar to remove hip tension.
4. The cat pulling its tail—with a bolster to stretch the quadriceps.
5. *Bhujangasana*—the cobra pose.
   After a few weeks of therapy, you evaluate the status of your back, and you can then add these poses, if it is appropriate.
6. *Adho Mukha Svanasana*—the downward-facing dog pose
7. *Ustrasana*—the camel pose
8. *Savasana*—Meditation, with a bolster, to raise the upper body.

Add a visualization (see Chapter 9) during Savasana for feeling the back muscles in good health with their strength and flexibility.

The emotional symbolism of hernia and disc protrusion

Ask yourself why this happens to you. Of course, hernias and protrusions have mechanical causes, but keep in mind that the human being is a whole, including the body, the mind, and the emotions.

I often observe that people suffering from these pathologies feel they are trapped financially. Their relationship with money is not fluid; they care about it but do not contribute to its flow. The other possibility is that not enough money comes in, which creates the feeling of being trapped. They want to escape— leave this situation to feel free. It is possible to see a parallel between the disc abnormally leaving its envelope in which it was "prisoner" and the person looking to get out of a situation in which she feels prisoner. Most of the time, it is related to finances and material items.

Are you in a financially dependent situation? Or maybe you are in a relationship in which you feel captive, not up to par, or submissive?

A hernia and a protrusion are signs you must check. The healing process is through assertiveness and release from relationships in which you may have felt like a prisoner. The substance coming out of the disc or causing the disc to bulge can then subside, and with some patience, everything will be back to normal. Self-healing consists of working on your self confidence so you feel free! Dare to be autonomous and independent!

Sciatica

Sciatica is the usual name for sciatic nerve neuralgia. There are two sciatic nerves, and they are the biggest in the human body. They start behind the lumbar vertebrae and the sacrum, the pelvic region vertebrae, and extend to the toes. In general, sciatica only concerns the nerve, which is compressed, inflamed, or damaged. That causes tension and pain on the side of the buttock and down the leg, sometimes down to the toes. You can also feel tingling, numbness, or muscle weakness in the leg and foot.

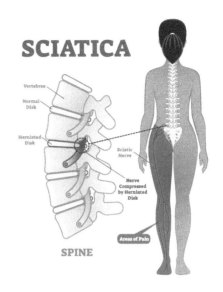

Among pregnant women, sciatica is often present about the sixteenth week. The weight of the belly, combined with increased secretion of a hormone, relaxin, that softens tissues, that press on the sciatic nerve.

Risk factors

- Practicing a sport or having a job requiring the lifting heavy loads.
- Curbing or making frequent torso torsions.
- Remaining seated for many continuous hours.
- Doing little physical activity.
- Being overweight.
- Weak abdominal muscles.

How to treat this problem

The goal is for you to get rid of this pain in the buttock area or the leg and remove the inflammation. To relax those regions, I suggest you practice the following Yin Yoga exercises.

Supta Kapotasana—the reclined pigeon pose to stretch the piriformis.

Supta Padangustasana—to stretch the hamstring.

Bhujangasana—the cobra pose.

Urdhva Svanasana—the upward facing dog pose.

Supta Baddha Konasana—the reclined butterfly with a bolster and belt.

Savasana – final relaxation with a bolster to elevate your upper back.

The emotional symbolism of sciatica

The emotional factors of sciatica relate to a physical block when you walk. The inflammatory pain prevents you from going forward as you would like. You feel that things do not go fast enough; everything is slow. This frustration can then be expressed in sciatica.

The pain symbolizes your incapacity to reach your goals in the desired time. Very often, it is routine that prevents you from progressing. Fear of change also plays a role, and often, you repeat the same schemes. You need to overcome this anxiety and dare to take another path to heal the sciatica. Your fear of not having enough material resources adds to the intensity.

Financial issues can intensify this problem, but they are different from those of a hernia: they indicate a fear of not

having enough funds to properly take care of your dependents.
A lack of confidence in your abilities makes you doubt your
capacity to take care of people that need it. This feeling blocks
you, like the sciatic nerve. Your body gives you signs to dare
you to change and get out of your routine. Remember that your
fears block the energy and that dwelling on negative thoughts
attracts the negative!

Piriformis syndrome

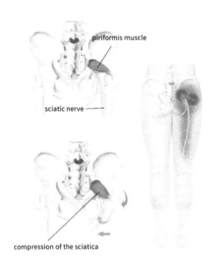

piriformis muscle

sciatic nerve

compression of the sciatica

The piriformis muscle extends
from sacrum's pelvic side to
the upper limit of the greater
trochanter of the femur. The
small and large buttocks
(*gluteus minimus* and *gluteus
maximus*) are superimposed
above it.

The buttocks are made
of three superficial muscles:
gluteus maximus, medius,
and *minimus*. Now called
gluteal muscles, they act
together to stabilize the pelvis and allow thigh movement. They
also stabilize the sacrum.

When you look at an anatomy chart, the *gluteus minimus*
and *maximus* are the largest muscles but don't consider the
piriformis less significant because it is smaller and deeper. It is
a hip adductor when the hip is in flexion and an external rotator
when it is in extension. It also stabilizes the sacrum and hip
during movement. A medical diagnosis is required to determine
if a piriformis syndrome exists. This examination involves
controlling pain in the buttocks during an internal rotation of
the thigh and during an abduction.

While running or sitting, the piriformis can compress the sciatic nerve, where it emerges under the piriformis and passes over the hip rotating muscles. You can then have sciatica because the liquid from the hernia touches the nerve and inflames it or because the piriformis irritates it.

Extremes are rarely healthy; it is thus not surprising that the piriformis syndrome happens to assiduous athletes as well as sedentary people. Remaining seated also leads to the atrophy of that muscle responsible for pain in the buttocks, legs, and toes. This pain is chronic and worsens with a sedentary lifestyle or heavy sporting demands.

Risk Factors

- Weak quadriceps.
- Running or frequent walking.
- A sedentary lifestyle.
- Repetitive movement.
- A trauma, like an injury or a fall.

How to Treat this Problem

Practice the following poses for relief. All these movements flex and abduct the hip. I suggest you do, in order:

1. *Rajakapotasana*—the king pigeon pose
2. *Supta Kapotasana*—the reclined pigeon pose
3. *Agnistambhasana*—the fire log pose
4. *Mandukasana*—the frog pose.

The emotional symbolism of the piriformis syndrome

The piriformis in the buttocks one of the deepest muscular layers. Note that those muscles allow you to go forward. Does this syndrome appear to force you to rest? You are not listening enough to your body and mind. During sciatic nerve inflammation because of the piriformis, you are forced to stop and heal yourself. Running, walking, and many other forms of physical activity relieve the piriformis and can let you escape. Sometimes, it can be necessary to face your problem. On the other hand, however, if you suffer from this syndrome because you have too sedentary a lifestyle, it may be connected to the fact you might feel forced to stay seated in your place. You do not dare to get up and leave your current position. The powerless feeling settles in. You then feel useless while being seated, but something stops you. Why not get up? Dare to assert yourself and move!

I suggest meditating on the subject to keep listening to the ideas that come up, so you can analyze them and act.

Sacroiliac joint injury

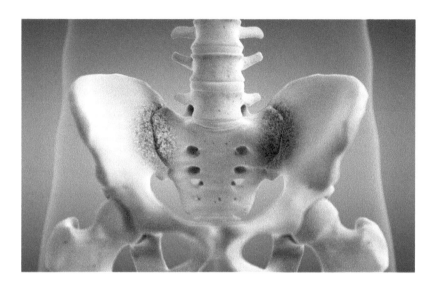

This is about two joints between the pelvic bones (iliac bone, coccyx, and sacrum) at the bottom of the spine, making the shape of a pivot. This sacroiliac joint is not very mobile, moving only a little when you move and walk. When it blocks, you can feel local pain in your lower back, in the buttocks, and sometimes down the leg. This discomfort can be on only one side or both. A medical diagnosis is required to distinguish a sacroiliac joint injury from a hernia. The pain can cause low back pain and become chronic.

Many researchers refer to sacroiliac joint injury during pregnancy. It seems to be linked to various factors. Posture changes causing hyperlordosis and weakness of the abdominal strap promote lower back and sacroiliac pain. Added to that are the hormonal changes: the ligaments become softer to allow this joint more mobility, possibly leading to painful instability and blockage.

Risk Factors

- Hyperlaxity and pregnancy hormonal changes.
- Traumas: like a fall from a height.
- Hypermobility from heredity.
- Degenerative injuries: like arthrosis.
- Inflammations: like ankylosing spondylitis, or inflammatory bowel disease.

How to treat this condition

I suggest you do the following poses when you feel light pain, but also when you feel no pain at all, because they are also preventive.

1. Begin with Matsyendrasana—the seated twist pose. If you are at ease, you can put the arm between the calf and the thigh, then cross fingers or catch the wrist to intensify the torsion

2. Add Jathara Parivartanasana—the reclining twist pose

If you want to try a variation, cross the right leg over the left, then turn towards the left, looking in the other direction.

The emotional symbolism of a sacroiliac joint injury

The sacrum region (pelvic region) is linked to sexuality and reproduction, the strongest energies in that region. The second chakra, Svatisthana, originates there.

If you have pain in this articulation, it could be a matter of sexual devaluation. Maybe you do not feel up to it, or not feel desirable or sexy. Your soul can express that through this injury. Since those tensions can turn into chronic lower back pain, you need to consider that the lumbar region also relates to money and responsibility. Are you running away from your financial obligations? Maybe you do not dare to go forward. Have trust in yourself and your destiny. Everything happening to you makes you grow!

I often note that confidence in oneself and assertiveness progressively reduce pain from a sacroiliac injury. Take responsibility for your life and welcome changes.

Stenosis

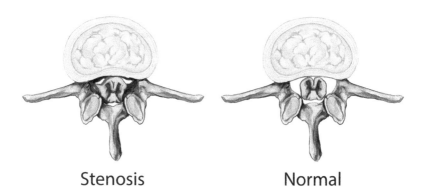

Stenosis   Normal

Spinal stenosis is caused by the narrowing of the spinal canal and can occur at different levels of the spine. It is often found in the cervical region (C5-C6 and C6-C7), the lumbar region (L4-L5), and the lumbar-sacrum region (L5-S1). A reduction of the diameter of that canal can lead to irritation of the spinal cord or nerve roots. This degenerative condition causes pain in the lower back region and lower limbs. You can then have problems walking, tingling sensations, or heavy legs.

The spinal cord's function is to transmit messages between the brain and the rest of the body. Spinal stenosis can thus have neurological consequences. As a result, you can get quickly tired while walking, and feel a general weakness in your lower body.

Risk factors

- Arthrosis
- Discal hernia
- Vertebral trauma (for example, a broken bone)
- Congenital condition (at birth)
- Scoliosis
- Spondylolisthesis.

How to treat stenosis

Over the long term, certain therapy postures efficiently relieve stenosis symptoms. This includes the strengthening of the legs, back, and abdominals.

When walking, you can plan pauses to prevent early fatigue, and add the following postures:

1. *Bhujangasana*, the cobra pose, and *Urdhva Mukha Svanasana*, the upward facing dog pose: to relieve the cervical vertebrae. It helps to lift your chin while inhaling and lower it while exhaling. This neck extension and flexion mobilize the neck and maintain its flexibility and agility

2. *Paschimottanasana*—the caterpillar: you can use a cushion to make this posture more accessible

3. *Navasana*—the boat pose: to reinforce the core of the body

4. *Supta Padangustasana* A, B & C—stretching the hamstrings.

The emotional symbolism of stenosis

Stenosis narrows the spinal canal at different locations on the spine. This canal sits behind the vertebrae, which protect the spine and gives it stability. Pain caused by the reduction of this canal within the dorsal vertebrae can symbolize a lack of confidence and security. You suffer from a lack of affection. It is possible that you do not find the stability you seek in your intimate relationships and that you lack confidence in yourself.

If the stenosis appears in the cervical vertebrae, that is often a sign of an inability to express your emotions. You talk a lot, but never about deep subjects, and sometimes say nothing.

Stenoses from the lumbar regions can show a lack of financial stability in your life. The five lumbar vertebrae are in a spot responsible for anchoring and rooting. It is possible that you feel you are not in your place, not sure of what you want in life. A certain fear related to material things comes back regularly and saddens you.

Visualize your life being full of abundance, surrounded by people who support you and who ensure a safe and stable environment.

How Yin Yoga can relieve muscular back pain

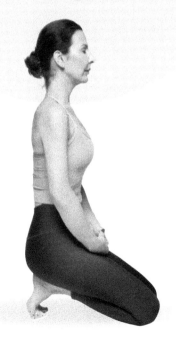

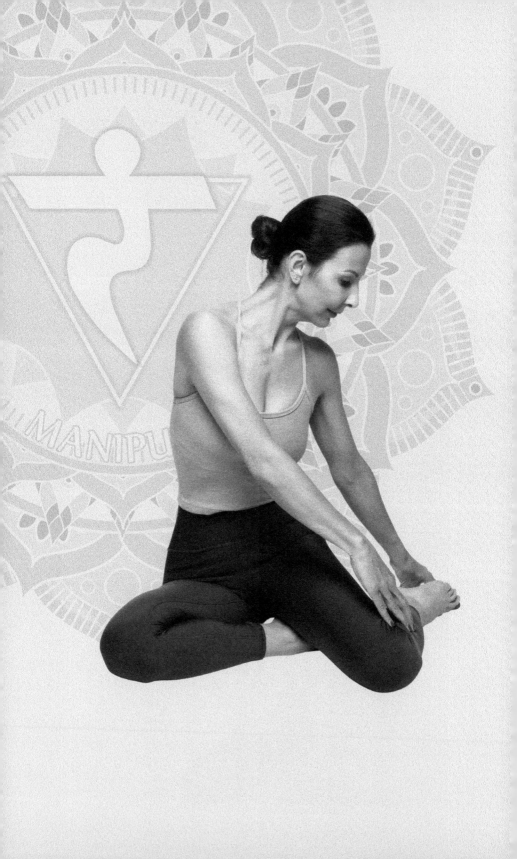

O ur body needs to move to stay flexible and produce synovial fluid. This is the liquid present in the joint spaces. It is both transparent and viscous, and its consistency is close to raw egg white. It is generated by the tissue cells lining the joint (the synovium). Its major role is to

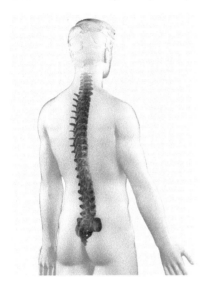

ensure joint lubrication, but it also feeds the cartilage and the cells to reduce the wear of the joint surfaces during friction. Spending most of your time seated, without moving, can lead to a lack of flexibility and arthrosis.

For your physical and mental health, it is essential to move so the energy can flow around, and to ensure nutrition and lubrication to your joints.

Sitting, a factor in malnutrition of the intervertebral discs

A functional spine has two physiological lordoses: cervical and lumbar. In a seated position, those curves disappear, and the lumbar lordosis is erased, even inverted, because the posture is arched. The cervical lordosis compensates by increasing its radius. Discs are pinched forward, and the back ligaments are stretched. Besides that, there is an absence of vascularization within the intervertebral disc, which is submitted to friction forces and elevated, continuous pressures. Elimination of waste is thus carried out by a simple circulation within the vertebrae.

The disc deflates when it is compressed and fills up when it is relaxed in a lying position, for example. These liquid exchanges constantly function during life's daily activities and allow the disc to be nourished. Body movement and position changes, in some way, ensure the health of the disc over time.

So staying in a seated position for a long time does not favor the nourishment of the intervertebral discs, while moving between seated and standing positions, as well as physical exercises, contributes to providing energy to the disc and delaying its aging. Making changes in your daily life, like buying a stand-up desk or moving regularly, can save your joints and your back.

It is unnecessary to practice high-intensity activities to produce synovial fluid and correctly nourish your joints. Try, for example, the following Yin postures (see explanations of the poses in Chapter VIII) and your pain will go away.

- *Uttanasana*—standing forward fold, with stretched and bent knees.
- *Baddha Konasana*—the butterfly.
- *Janu Sirsasana*—head on knee pose.
- *Paschimottanasana*—the caterpillar.
- *Utthan Pristhasana*—the lizard pose.
- *Urdhva Mukha Svanasana*—the upward facing dog pose.
- *Bhujangasana*—the cobra pose.
- *Jathara Parivartanasana*—the reclining twist pose.
- *Savasana*—final relaxation, with or without bolster.

Pathologies connected to rheumatism

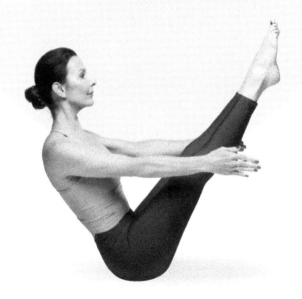

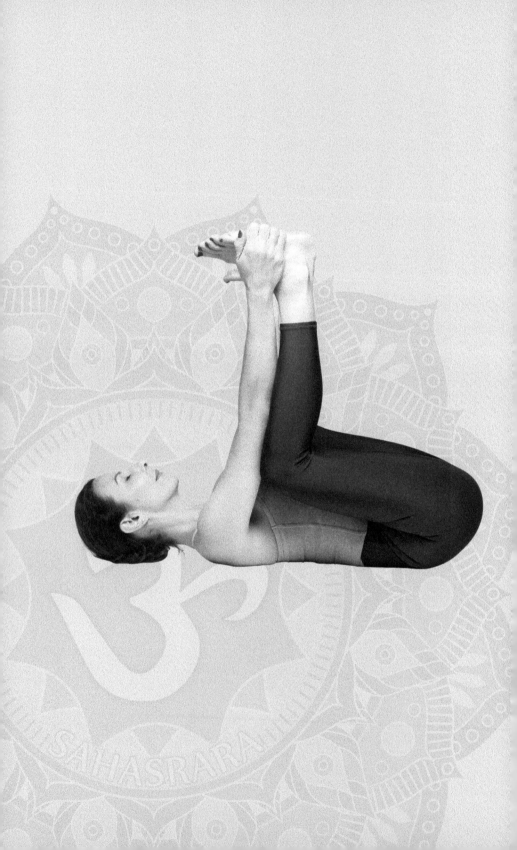

Rheumatism generally designates all mechanical pathologies of the locomotor system that impact joints. It can be damage to cartilage, the synovial membrane, the tendon, or an intervertebral disc. It is also possible to talk of arthrosis, arthritis, osteoporosis, or autoimmune diseases like rheumatoid arthritis. These disorders can cause some chronic pain. However, my experience shows that when you integrate regular movements and relaxation into your daily routine, you can relieve that pain. Often, the pain goes away when the joint is warmed up. Otherwise, you simply adapt and change the movement's execution to avoid any tension.

Arthrosis or arthritis - what is the difference?

Both conditions come from the family of rheumatism; the common symptom is joint pain. Arthrosis is a mechanical condition characterized by the gradual wear of joint cartilage. Aging and wear are the two most common risk factors for it. With advanced arthrosis, joint bones rub against each other, causing major pain and a loss of mobility. A waking-up pain is, for example, a typical characteristic, but symptoms disappear soon after you wake as you begin to move. It is thus essential to practice regular stretching exercises to fight back the loss of flexibility and agility.

Arthritis is not caused by normal bone wear. Rather, it is an inflammation caused by the secretion of substances gradually destroying the joint structure. It is more intense at rest, especially during the night. You will generally notice a warm sensation near the affected joint, as well as redness and swelling, and is often noticed in fingers. It can be of infectious, genetic, or metabolic origin. Arthritis often appears between the ages of 40 and 60.

Arthrosis risk factors

- Aging.
- Certain physical jobs, with repetitive movements especially for wrists and elbows.
- High-frequency sports practice: all the joints involved could be problematic.
- Obesity, overweight: this often affects knees and hips.
- Lack of exercise.

Arthritis risk factors

- Hereditary aspects.
- An immune disorder.

Ankylosing spondylitis

Ankylosing spondylitis is another form of inflammatory rheumatism and is more frequent among men than women. It mostly affects the spine and the pelvis. With time, the dorsal vertebrae intertwine, and the spine may stiffen. Some patients cannot turn their heads because of the numbness of their cervical vertebrae. In other cases, they lose mobility in the lumbar region, reducing their forward and backward mobility.

Systemic inflammatory diseases are the most common conditions nowadays resulting from this pathology. Inflammations appear not only among joints but also within organs.

Abarticular rheumatisms

As indicated by their name, abarticular rheumatisms are mostly rheumatisms that do not affect joints. There are some pathologies like fibromyalgia (diffuse muscle pain and tenderness), periarthritis (inflammation of the tissues surrounding the joint), tendinitis (inflammation of the tendons), and bursitis (inflammation of the bursae).

How to treat abarticular rheumatism

Theoretically, there is no treatment for those rheumatisms, but I suggest you do the following exercises to relieve the pain and maintain your flexibility and strength at least twice a week. I often notice that my clients are living with this type of problem without being particularly bothered, thanks to their practicing relaxing positions.

The best treatment is a mix of cardiovascular exercises (like walking, cycling, and swimming), muscular strengthening exercises, and relaxation exercises. Staying at least three minutes in Yin Yoga poses allows you to stretch deeply to the tendons and fasciae in order to establish and maintain functional flexibility and have a better quality of life.

I suggest you do a session including all the spine movements possible: flexions, extensions, and rotations, with the goal of creating physical harmony and maintaining general flexibility for living without pain and tension.

1. *Adho Mukha Svanasana*—the downward-facing dog pose, with accessories, if you want them.
2. *Parsva Vajrasana*—the thunderbolt pose.
3. P*aschimottanasana*—the caterpillar, with the bolster variant if it is more comfortable.
4. *Bhujangasana*—the cobra pose.

5. *Supta Padangustasana A, B & C*—to stretch the hamstrings.

6. *Mandukasana*—the frog pose.

7. *Savasana*—final relaxation, with a bolster.

The emotional symbolism of rheumatism

Articular and abarticular rheumatisms can cause some pain and some rigidity. Here are some key analytical points illustrating the connection between body, mind, and emotions based on a study case. I will never forget my meeting with this client suffering from arthrosis, arthritis, and fibromyalgia over ten years ago. She came to see me to gain flexibility to get rid of her pain. She added that she was aware of her rigidity, both on the physical and mental levels, and noticed it daily in both her personal and professional lives. This clarity surprised me. I frequently observe parallels between personality traits and the physical aspects of my clients, but it is rare that a client has such acute awareness. This person was far from having functional flexibility. Considering her emotions and her physiological needs, we established sessions to untie those in both areas. The work on her body and mind, as well as the confidence we built between ourselves, contributed to the disappearance of her chronic pain.

It has been proven that stress can cause rheumatism. The hormones produced by stress (like cortisol) contribute to bone destruction. I suggest you write down the elements that could stress you or upset you. Why are you becoming rigid? But, especially, what could you do so you don't feel the need (consciously or not) to be rigid? Take the time to do this exercise for many consecutive days, then analyze the results. Carry out the flexibility exercises in parallel and meditate on your life's physical and psychological flexibility.

I am convinced you can learn to manage and get rid of these unpleasant conditions. Become more flexible in your body and mind!

Bursitis

Bursitis is an inflammation of the parts that the support and act as a junction between the bones and tendons. It is characterized by inflammation and swelling in a bursa and is usually very painful. The bursa is like a bag filled with liquid located under the skin. Bursae secrete a lubricant fluid to reduce friction between the various mobile parts of the joint and, that way, prevent arthrosis. The most frequent bursitises appear around the hips, knees, shoulders, and elbows.

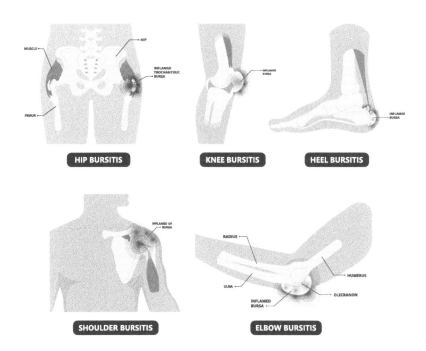

Bursitis Risk Factors

- Repeating an effort.
- A micro-traumatis.
- An unusual movement of a joint.
- The use and prolonged pressure on the affected limb.
- Arthritis.
- A bad posture.

Shoulder Bursitis

The glenohumeral joint is the most flexible in the body; it can perform flexions, extensions, abductions, adductions, and forward and backward pushes, as well as internal and external rotations. When a risk factor is present, over-secretion causes bursa inflammation. A shoulder bursitis is often accompanied by pain related to movements of the joint or tendons. Indeed, those movements worsen the inflammation, perpetuating the problem. The smallest daily gesture, like putting clothes on or simply sleeping, can be painful. We must not forget that this pain is simply a sign that we should avoid certain moves.

Later, I will give you some poses to strengthen the rotator cuff in the shoulder, which includes muscles and tendons connecting the humerus to the scapula, and to stabilize the shoulder girdle, the bone structure connecting the torso and the shoulder.

To go further, let us analyze the anatomy of this glenohumeral joint.

The shoulder comprises bones, ligaments, tendons, and muscles to connect the arm and the torso. As you can see in the illustration below, the articulation is formed by three bones: clavicle, scapula, and humerus. The shoulder has two joints allowing the arm to move.

The acromioclavicular joint is an orbicular joint between the clavicle and the acromion and allows us to lift the arm above

the head. The acromion is an extension of the scapula, forming
the extremity of the shoulder.

The glenohumeral joint is a mobile joint. Its head,
corresponding to the spherical end of the humerus, fits into the
concave part of the scapula, called the glenoid cavity. Thanks to
this joint, the arm can do circles as well as movements in front
the body.

The four muscles of the rotator cuff maintain the humerus
against the scapula. Those muscles allow stabilizing the
glenohumeral joint and to move the arms in circular motions.
Because of the great mobility of this joint and the belonging of
the rotator cuff to deep muscular layers, injuries and tears can
often occur.

- The rotator cuff comprises many muscles (SIST)
- Supraspinatus
- Infraspinatus
- Subscapularis
- Teres minor

Shoulder Anatomy

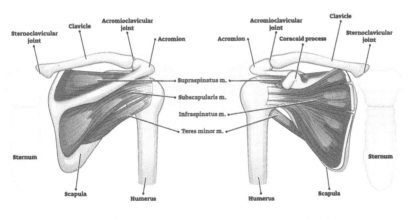

Posterior view   Anterior view

Shoulder bursitis risk factors

- Repetitive movements.
- Physiologically incorrect alignments.
- Rotator cuff underdeveloped muscles.
- Instability and hyperlaxity of the glenohumeral girdle.

How to treat shoulder bursitis

To relieve bursitis pain, you first need to avoid painful movements, strengthen the rotator cuff, and perform some exercises to stabilize the shoulder girdle.

I suggest, for example, the following exercises:

1. Hold the elastic in your hands. Position the right elbow at the hip with the elbow bent at 90°. The other hand holds the elastic and does not move. Inhale while pulling on the elastic with the right hand and keeping the elbow bent at 90° against the hip. Do 10 repetitions on each side.

   Note: Hold the elastic while placing both elbows at 90° on each hip. Inhale while pulling away both hands, then exhale while returning to the initial position.

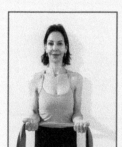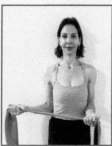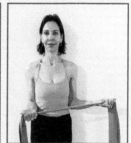

2. You can follow up with *Adho Mukha Svanasana*—the downward-facing dog pose to strengthen the shoulder girdle.

3. *Mandukasana*—the frog pose to stabilize shoulders.

4. *Salabhasana*—the grasshopper pose to strengthen the posterior deltoid.

5. *Parsva Vajrasana*—the thunderbolt, with or without rotation to maintain joint flexible and to avoid calcification.

6. Finally, *Supta Baddha Konasana*— the reclined butterfly to open your posture and increase your pulmonary capacity.

The emotional symbolism of the shoulder

You carry loads on your shoulders that cause you pain. Joys, sorrows, and responsibilities can represent a heavy weight. It is possible that some things upset you and are expressed as chronic tension in this area.

The weight of life seems too heavy to carry, and this emotional load becomes oppressive. I suggest you ease your daily life and refocus on yourself. Requesting help can be useful to free yourself from that pain. You do not need to carry all the world's misery on your shoulders. Dare to change and integrate more lightness in your life.

I remember a client who told me about her sessions with her hypnotherapist, during which she had to express her physical sensations for more than an hour. She found that boring until, a few hours after her sessions, she felt tension and a significant load on her shoulders. She then realized that was connected to the responsibilities while taking care of her sick mom and being a single mom. She practiced some therapeutic yoga poses and hired a nurse to have more time with her children. A few weeks later, she came to see me again, and her pain had disappeared.

Knee bursitis

Thanks to the knee joint, you can do flexions and extensions.

It's a good idea to distinguish between acute and chronic bursitis. Acute bursitis develops in a few hours only, maybe over a few days. Like shoulder bursitis, knee bursitis causes pain when you move or touch the area. The surrounding skin may be red and swollen.

I suffered from many acute knee bursitises after my ACL (anterior cruciate ligament) and meniscus surgery. That was the result of practicing exercises too intensely. The solution was for the sports doctor to remove the excess liquid. Normally, this liquid is beneficial for your joints but, when too much is produced, it can cause major pain. Chronic bursitis can result from repeated or continual acute bursitises or trauma. If the bursae are altered or submitted to an unusual exercise or tension, the inflammation can worsen. If that lasts for too much time, pain and swelling can limit the movement and weaken the muscle structure. Cases of chronic bursitis can last for months and return.

Anatomy of the knee

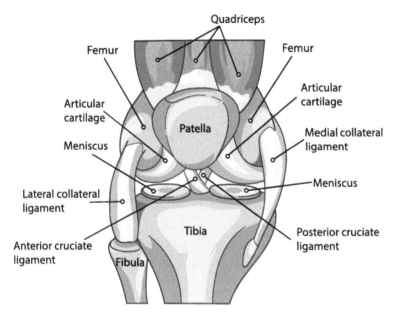

The knee is formed by three bone parts:

1. The lower end of the femur: the condyles.
2. The upper end of the tibia: the tibial plateau.
3. The patella (small shield on the front of the femur).

There are also other elements helping the complex function of the joint:

■ A cartilage layer, covering each bone: the femoral condyles, anterior part of the femur, posterior side of the patella and the tibial plateau.

■ Two small cushions of fibrous cartilage, the menisci, between the femur and the tibia, are shaped like croissants. They absorb the contact between the femur and tibia's cartilages. One is located on the outside (the medial or internal meniscus), and the other is on the inside of the knee (lateral or external meniscus).

- Two cruciate ligaments (CL) ensure joint stability: an anterior cruciate ligament (ACL) going from top to bottom, front to back and outside to inside, and a posterior cruciate ligament (PCL) going from top to bottom, back to front, inside to outside to form a hinge inside the knee. The ACL crosses the PCI laterally, as you can see from the illustration.

- Two collateral ligaments (tibial or internal and fibular or external) support the knee, inside and outside. They also cross, allowing good knee stability.

- Ligaments support the patella, the patellar or patellar tendon; quadriceps to the tibia, even during a knee flexion; the patella to the tibia and tendons of the quadriceps muscle, linking the patella to the thigh. They ensure the transmission of the traction of the quadriceps to the tibia, even during serious knee inflexions, with the patella acting like a pulley.

- A joint capsule containing synovial fluid to bathe the inside of the joint and promotes sliding.

Knee bursitis risk factors

- Repetitive movements.
- Excessive exercises.
- A rehabilitation that is too intense and does not respect the recovery stages.

How to treat a knee bursitis

To heal a knee bursitis, you first need to rest. It is a painful inflammation, indicating that you need to listen to your body and take time to rest. To maintain certain flexibility and mental well-being, I suggest you soften the muscles around the knee to avoid unnecessary tension arising from immobilization.

You can begin with:

1. *Adho Mukha Svanasana*—the downward-facing dog pose
2. *Paschimottanasana*—the caterpillar, with the support of a bolster, if needed
3. *Maksikanagasana*—The Dragonfly Pose
4. the wide angle seated forward bend pose, with an optional bolster
5. *Supta Padangustasana* A, B & C—stretching the hamstrings
6. *Halasana*—the plow pose
7. *Karnapidasana*—the ear pressure pose
8. *Viparita Karana*—the supine position with legs lifted.

Applying ice and refreshing creams can also be useful.

The emotional symbolism of a knee bursitis

What is that knee pain trying to tell you? The knee is essential for bending and going forward, which can remind us that we kneel at church to seek forgiveness. The fluid in this joint represents your anger towards a person seeking to play an authoritarian role, which upsets you. The inflammation expresses your refusal of such behavior from a person around you. Can you see how that is connected to what is happening around you?

I suggest you look inside to see what makes you feel good. Focus on your quintessence and keep listening to what you would like to happen in your life.

Give less importance to others, and keep in mind that you can only influence your own emotions. Remind yourself that you cannot change others, nor what happens to you, but you can change how you react. Your attitude will determine your character and destiny.

Hip bursitis

The hip is a very mobile joint, like the shoulder. It can perform flexions, extensions, abductions, adductions, and forward and backward rotations.

Hip bursitis is a common problem in orthopedics. It is expressed by pain on the external side of the thigh and hip, resulting from inflammation of a bursa around the hip, a little pocket filled with synovial fluid for lubricating the space between the tendons and bones to ease movement.

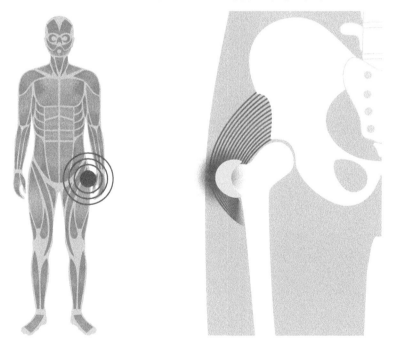

There are many bursae in the hips that could be the origin of bursitis, but trochanteric bursitis is the most common. The trochanter is a bony prominence on the hips outside where the tendons connect.

The hip is a coxo-femoral joint between the femur (thigh bone) and the coxal bone (iliac bone) at the pelvis level. The femur has a head and a neck in the upper part. The head articulates in the acetabulum, the articular cavity of the coxal bone. The head and the cavity are covered in cartilage about 3mm thick. The acetabulum is also surrounded by fibrocartilage, the acetabulum labrum.

The most common pathologies are arthrosis and bursitises.

Hip Bursitis Risk Factors

- A traumatism, like a fall, for example
- Exercises with repetitive impacts
- Chronic joint overload.

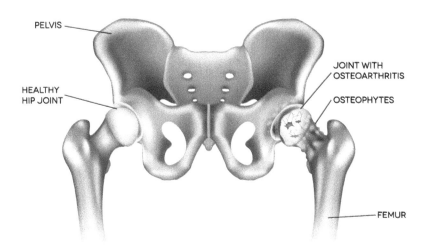

Hip joint osteoarthritis

How to treat this problem - Just as for the shoulder and the knee, it's a good idea to consider the inflammation and pain and prevent any movement that could cause discomfort. However, it is important to keep the joint mobile and flexible. I suggest you start with:

1. Marjarasana—the cat pose to move the hip and the spine.
2. Supta Kapotasana—the reclined pigeon pose.
3. Rajakapotasana—the pigeon, moving slowly and paying attention to the tension, and adapting the amplitude of the movement, if necessary.
4. Navasana—the boat pose to tone the center of the body.
5. Salabhasana—the grasshopper pose to strengthen the posterior muscles.
6. Viparita Karana—the lying down position with legs raised, using a wall as support.
7. Halasana—the plow pose.
8. Karnapidasana—the ear pressure pose to invert gravity and remove weight from the hips.

The emotional symbolism of the hip

The hip joint is symbolic of going forward. Bursitis, or another rheumatoid illness, can prevent you from walking. What message does your body transmit to you this way? Do you fear change? Does your hip slow you because you do not dare to jump?

The hip supports you. Are you angry with someone who does not support you as you wish? Can you no longer move forward because that situation is becoming unbearable?

The inflammation is a stop sign, and it helps you to take time to rest. Maybe it is time to face the situation or the person causing this problem. To speed along the self-healing path, give yourself the tools to make changes in your life. Dare to jump!

The energy system: the chakras

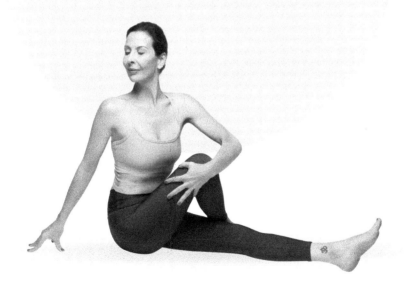

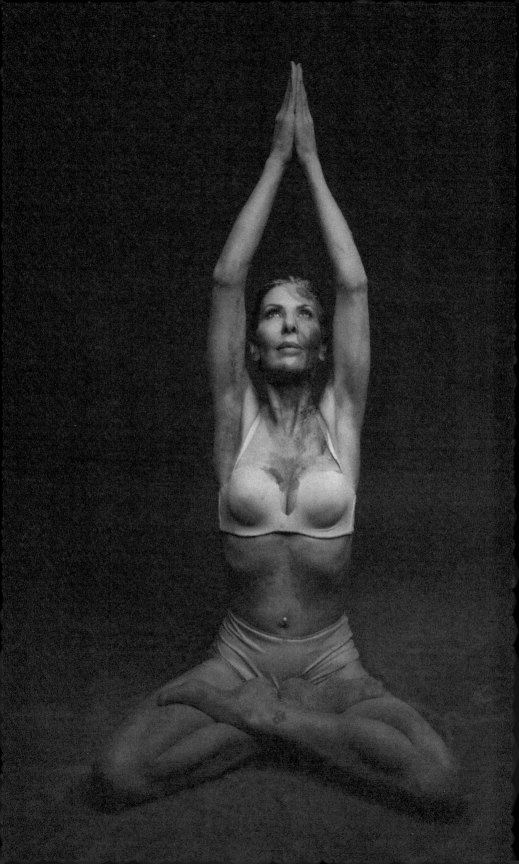

Chakra comes from Sanskrit and means either "wheel" or "disc." Chakras identify connecting points between the physical body and the astral body, a person's invisible energy envelope. Those energy centers are responsible for your vitality, as well as your physical and mental well-being. They are along the spine, from the perineum to the skull. A chakra is like a magnetic node on your physical body.

The two *nadis* (energy canals), *ida* and *pingala*, are wrapped around the spine, *sushumna*, and thus form the chakras, allowing Prana, the vital energy, to flow around.

Sushumna means "the main psychic route" in Tantric yoga philosophy. It is one of the three *nadis*. *Sushumna* is the central canal passing through the spine, at the origin of *kundalini*, vital energy flowing along the chakras. Together with *ida* and *pingala*, they form something like a caduceus (the symbol with two serpents entwined around a sword).

The *ida* originates on the spine's left, at the Muladhara Chakra's level, and rolls up around *the sushumna* like the *pingala*. *Ida* corresponds to lunar energy, Yin, the feminine principle.

The *pingala* originates on the spine's right of the spine, at the Muladhara Chakra level, and rolls up, around the *sushumna* like the *ida*. *Pingala* corresponds to solar energy, Yang, the masculine principle.

Chakras and energy channels

When these energy centers work perfectly, they represent spinning wheels whose color is dazzling. If a chakra is unsettled, the wheel spins more slowly and the color fades, which can lead to negative mental, emotional, and physical consequences.

The chakras develop in cycles at precise moments in life, starting in the mother's womb. Childhood up to the age of 7 is considered an especially significant phase. Traumatic events such as a lack of love, parental indifference, and repression of

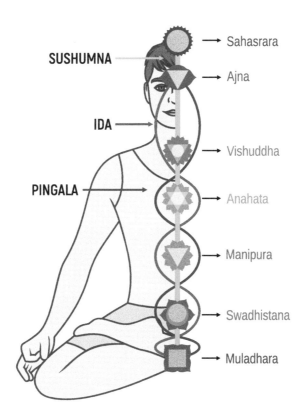

natural needs can lead to the incorrect development of some chakras. So, the first year of life is especially influential for the *Muladhara* chakra, responsible for the original trust. If the newborn is separated from its mother, or its needs of warmth and food are not satisfied, this can lead to an absence of trust and to existential fears in the adult. Other traumatic events or a lifestyle in disagreement with your quintessence can cause a blockage of chakras that were previously well developed. Some emotions, like fear, envy, pride, or hatred, can cause those blockages, just as can an exaggerated conformism, added to the suppression of emotions.

Each of the seven chakras is considered an energy node, connected not only to the physical body but also to the soul and the mind. One goal of Yin Yoga is to heal the body, the mind, and the soul, from an energy perspective and to find unity and serenity that was lost, so we can continue our spiritual development.

You find below an image representing the chakras and their color.

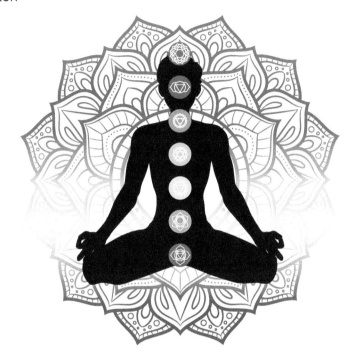

The chakras and their colors

1. Root Chakra—*Muladhara:* base of the spine, red

2. *Svadhishthana* Chakra—under the belly button, orange

3. Solar Plexus Chakra—*Manipura:* stomach area, yellow

4. Heart Chakra—*Anahata:* middle of the chest, green

5. Throat Chakra—*Vishuddha:* base of the throat, blue

6. Third Eye Chakra—*Aina:* forehead, between the eyes, indigo

7. Sacral Chakra/Crown Chakra—*Sahasrara:* top of the head, violet

The Chakras, their Functions and Promoting their Proper Functioning

1. *Muladhara* - Root chakra
Utthan Pristhasana the lizard pose

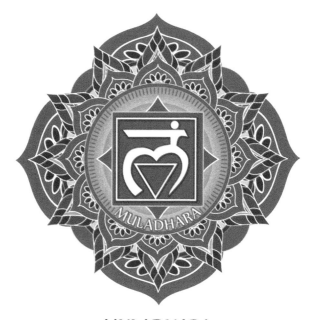

MULADHARA
Sanskrit: मूलाधार

ROOT CHAKRA

The Muladhara chakra is at the basis of the spine, at the root of the *kundalini* energy. It goes up along the *sushumna* to the seventh chakra, *sahasrara*. Red is the color of this energy center. It represents stability, rootedness, the force of nature, and internal harmony. This root chakra is in connection with the earth element, hence its sense of anchorage.

This is where personal and spiritual growth originates. Daring new experiences and asserting yourself, being confident in life and destiny are connected to it. Its functioning is strongly influenced by childhood. To have lived the first years of your life filled with love and devotion and not feel unmet primary needs has a fundamental effect on the rest of your life. This is how you develop and cultivate general confidence in life and in the people around you.

The presence of existential worries is a consequence of a malfunction of this energy center. The fear of not being able to satisfy basic needs, like being able to eat correctly or live in a safe and enjoyable location, is part of it.

The *kundalini* originates here. When you are a child, a snake, a symbol of vital energy leading to illumination, climbs along *sushumna*, the spine. It lives and retires here. When the kundalini wakes up, it climbs and brings you personal and spiritual enlightenment.

How to promote the proper functioning of the *muladhara* chakra

- Be aware of traumas you possibly experienced during childhood.
- Work with a psychologist, for example, on those negative events.
- Feel your body, do exercises, massages, and Yin Yoga to connect yourself.
- Walk in nature to feel Prana, the vital energy.

2. *Svadhishthana* - Sacral Chakra - *Jathara Parivartanasana* - The Reclining Twist Pose

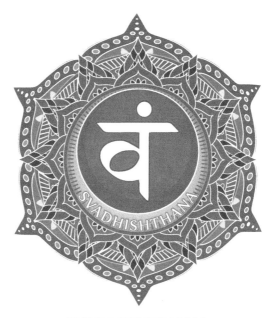

SVADHISHTHANA
Sanskrit: स्वाधिष्ठान

SACRAL CHAKRA

This chakra, located just below the belly button, controls the function of your sexual organs.

The Svadhishthana chakra radiates orange. Its element is water, and it represents the force of life, creativity, and passion. Your emotions are expressed and lived through it. If its functioning is not disturbed, you are full of self-esteem and can express and live your emotions without being ashamed on the sentimental and physical levels. You also live instinctively and easily express your needs.

How to promote the proper functioning of the Svadhishthana chakra

- Be aware of disturbing and traumatic events from your childhood and teenage years so you can work on them.
- Express your sensuality, by dancing, being creative, or through your sexuality.
- Review which subject or situation makes you feel ashamed and find out why.
- Stimulate the water element: keep well hydrated, swim, walk along water (a lake or ocean, for example).

3. *Manipura* - Solar Plexus Chakra
Bananasana - Banana Position

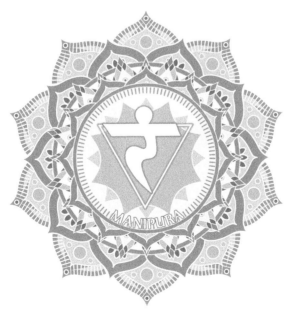

MANIPURA

Sanskrit: मणिपूर

SOLAR PLEXUS CHAKRA

The *Manipura* chakra is located towards the upper stomach and radiates yellow. Its element is fire. It represents your strength of character and will and your internal convictions, as well as your personality. This chakra is connected to your need to succeed; the idea of growing and developing more is also part of it.

An open *Manipura* chakra means you have a mature and calm personality. You have been able to integrate your inner child and use your experiences to grow and become wiser. The self-healing skills you have developed can help you overcome life obstacles. You also can stay calm and focused, even in stressful situations.

How to promote the proper functioning of the *Manipura* chakra

- Let your doubts and pain surface; try to understand why you are feeling them.
- Tap into your beliefs and ask if they can give direction to your life.
- Work with your inner child.
- Observe your fears and life obstacles, and face them.
- Do exercises for deep relaxation.
- Practice intense movements, like Vinyasa Yoga (dynamic yoga, based on the Yang principle).

4. *Anahata* - heart chakra
Anahatasana - the Puppy Dog Pose

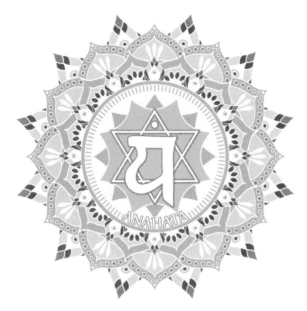

ANAHATA
Sanskrit: अनाहत

HEART CHAKRA

The *Anahata* chakra is around the heart, radiates green, and its element is the air. It represents love, empathy, and grateful and painful emotions.

If this chakra is open, you can love and be loved completely and unconditionally. You can do that only if you have enough self-esteem. To get there, you need to ignore the injuries of the previous three chakras, so you can give and receive. People around you feel that your heart chakra is open because you radiate happiness and love. You make yourself available to others and see your destiny linked to theirs to help and accompany them on their healing path.

How to promote the proper functioning of the *Anahata* chakra

- Become aware of things the way they are, and feel them accordingly
- Try to see love within yourself and others; dare to be vulnerable
- Forgive in order to be at peace with yourself and others
- Find your self-esteem to develop more love in your life.

5. *Vishuddha*—Throat Chakra *Ustrasana*—the Camel Pose

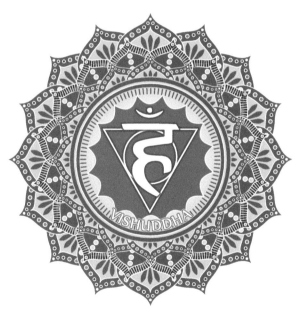

VISHUDDHA

Sanskrit: वशिुद्ध

THROAT CHAKRA

The *Vishuddha* chakra is at the throat level. It radiates sky blue, and its element is ether. This chakra influences your creativity and your ability to communicate.

If your throat chakra is open, you are a good listener and listen to others. You have a lot of empathy and thinking and know how to express various points of view clearly and accept your weak sides and live with them.

Some disturbing and traumatic events occurring between 16 and 21 can block the *Vishuddha* chakra. This can manifest through communication problems: you cannot verbalize what you feel, and you do not listen to others. There could be a tendency to lie frequently. Other people's opinions and reactions frighten you.

How to promote the proper functioning of the *Vishuddha* chakra

- Accept who you really are.
- Analyze the parts of your life where you are not sincere with yourself.
- Work on the acceptance of the imperfection in your life.
- Practice singing as a therapeutic tool.
- Speak in front of a group and express yourself.
- Observe your emotions when you have conversations.

6. Ajna - Third Eye chakra
Balasana - the Child's Pose

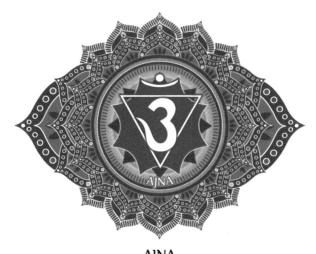

AJNA
Sanskrit: आज्ञा
THIRD-EYE CHAKRA

This chakra, found between the eyebrows, radiates royal blue and has spirit as its element. It represents intuition and wisdom. The third eye is connected with deep spirituality and makes you feel some energies.

In our society, the rational side connected to the brain's left side is central. However, this sixth energy center is often underdeveloped. Generally, people only begin to take time to develop their Ajna Chakra for spirituality and mysticism after the age of 21. It is connected with a potent release of energy and requires some maturity. You thus develop the ability to absorb those powerful energies.

How to promote the proper functioning of the *Ajna* chakra

- ▨ Do exercises to develop your intuition.
- ▨ Practice meditation and Pratyahara to take a step backward and know yourself better.
- ▨ Trust a superior force guiding you.
- ▨ Feel the waves.
- ▨ Trust your emotions.
- ▨ Practice creative visualization regularly (see Chapter 10, "Creative Visualization.")

7. *Sahasrara* - Crown Chakra *Padmasana* - the Lotus Pose

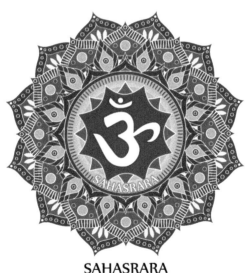

SAHASRARA

Sanskrit: सहस्रार

CROWN CHAKRA

The *Sahasrara* Chakra is on top of your head, has spirit as its element, and radiates violet. It expresses wisdom and major know-how.

If it is open, you live in a constant state of deep contentment. It opens when the *kundalini* goes up along the *sushumna*. The symbolic image is the snake twisting around the spine, leading to a state of liberation. You feel connected with the supreme energy and know that part of the universe is also part of you (the Atman-Braman principle of individual and universal conscience). You live with deep confidence and tolerance and feel deeply satisfied.

If you suffer from an identity crisis or no longer know who you are, you suffer from a blockage of the *Sahasrara* chakra.

How to promote the proper functioning of the *Sahasrara* chakra

- Ensure the lower chakras are functioning properly.
- Discover your spiritual side.
- Practice meditation.
- Believe in a superior force taking care of you.

Chakras are a teaching tool for explaining creative visualization meditation. This method, explained further in Chapter 10, helps you get to know yourself better so you can manifest what you really wish for in your life.

For your desires to become a reality, you need to define them. Then it's a good idea to meditate on the emotions you feel when you have what you want. This is a fundamental aspect of creative visualization: connect yourself with your emotions when your dreams become a reality. Those emotions manifest themselves in the first three chakras, *Muladhara, Manipura,* and *Svadistana.* They are related to anchorage, emotions, what is felt, the mind, the spirit, and the connection with the supreme. They determine your desires at the thought level rationally. For your desires to manifest, your rational thoughts, instinct, and emotions must meet in the middle, in the Anahata Chakra, the heart chakra.

For creative visualization to work, the chakras must work in synergy with your desires. You need to unite the intellect and instinct, the rational and abstract.

How the meridians are stimulated by Yin practice

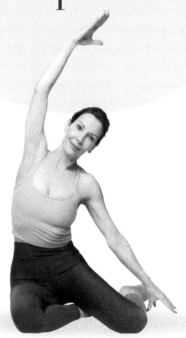

Chinese medicine, including acupuncture and Yin Yoga, works on the meridians. A meridian is an energy canal without corporal existence. That means you cannot touch it, but it exists on the astral level. It is a line connecting one point to another. The good working of the organs is connected to the meridians; by touching a meridian, you act on a precise organ.

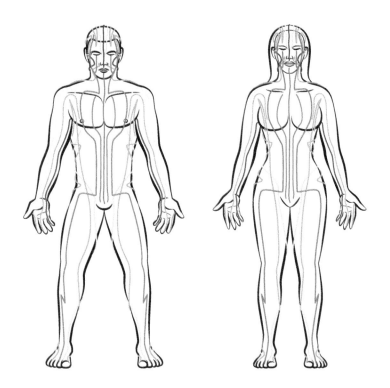

12 meridians

The 12 meridians are connected to the Yin and Yang system. Six are considered Yang, as they are connected to Yang organs:

- ◼ the large intestine.
- ◼ the stomach.
- ◼ the small intestine.

- the bladder.
- the gallbladder.
- the triple heater.

The other six are Yin, because they are connected to Yin organs:

- the lungs.
- the spleen.
- the heart.
- the kidneys.
- the liver.
- the pericardium.

If enough Chi passes through the meridians, they function well, and you enjoy very good health. In the opposite situation, your health could deteriorate.

The most common ways for making Chi flow around and avoid blockages are acupressure and acupuncture. The 365 acupuncture points act directly on those meridians located under the skin. It takes a full day for the Chi to cross all 12 meridians. The Yin and Yang meridians form couples. The Yin ones are located towards the center of the body and bring energy from the feet, crossing the center of the body, up to the fingers. The Yang ones are on the body's outside (skin surface) and bring energy from the fingers towards the face and the center of the body.

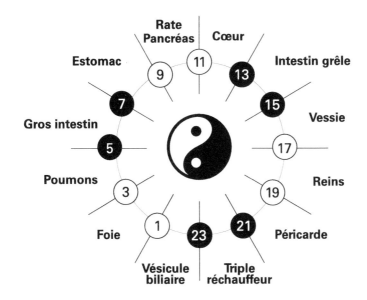

Each organ belongs to a precise schedule, and the Chi passes through each one for about two hours. If you regularly have a problem at a specific hour, it is highly probably linked to the malfunction of an organ.

- 01 AM – 03 AM = liver
- 03 AM – 05 AM = lungs
- 05 AM – 07 AM = colon
- 07 AM – 09 AM = stomach
- 09 AM – 11 AM = spleen
- 11 AM – 01 PM = heart
- 01 PM – 03 PM = small intestine
- 03 PM – 05 PM = bladder
- 05 PM – 07 PM = heart
- 09 PM – 11 PM = triple heater
- 11 PM – 01 AM = gallbladder

If you know that an organ is not working properly, I suggest you practice according to the time schedule. For example, in the case of a bladder problem, practice between 3 and 5 PM.

The Kidney Meridian

This Yin meridian goes from the middle of the sole of the foot to the calf, passing by the belly button, and ends below the clavicle. It belongs to the Sacral Chakra and symbolizes the root of life that blesses us with our existence.

It influences the birth and development of human beings. This meridian manages the energy reserves of our physical body and those we inherited from our parents. It is also responsible for our vitality and controls our hormonal distribution as well as our sexuality.

Troubles that can be linked to it include:

- bladder and kidney disease
- gynecological problems
- colds
- rheumatism
- fatigue
- fears and a certain pessimism.

Postures favoring the optimal function of the kidney meridian

1. Initial Meditation

I recommend the following mantra: repeat "energy" during each inhalation and "tension" during each exhalation. Then, visualize the energy entering your body, and all the tension will disappear.

2. Baddha Konasana—the butterfly

3. Bhujangasana—the cobra pose

4. Malasana—the garland pose

5. Ustrasana—the camel pose

6. Supta Virasana—the reclined hero pose

7. Savasana—final meditation.

   Maintain the poses for three minutes.

The Bladder Meridian

This Yang meridian passes from the third eye towards the head, then in the spine, along the back of the leg and ends outside the little toe (on both sides, of course). It also belongs to the Sacral Chakra. It regulates our nervous system and the balance of our bodily fluids. We need it to eliminate toxins. Problems that can be linked to it include:

- Nervous system diseases.
- Vertigo.
- Back pain.
- Tremors.
- Fever.
- Muscular pain.
- Stomach and colon diseases.
- Nervousness.

Postures favoring the optimal function of the bladder meridian

1. Baddha Konasana—the butterfly

2. Ustrasana—the camel pose

3. Balasana—the child's pose

4. Utthan Pristhasana—the lizard pose

5. Ananda Balasana—the happy baby pose

6. Malasana—the garland pose

7. Supta Virasana—the reclined hero pose

8. Bhujangasana—the cobra pose

9. Adho Mukha Svanasana—the downward-facing dog pose

10. Gomukasana—the cow face pose

11. Jathara Parivartanasana—the reclining twist pose

12. Halasana—the plow pose

The lung meridian

This Yin meridian passes under the collarbone towards the inside of the arm, then towards the thumb. It belongs to the Heart Chakra.

Its function is to transform the Chi in breath to maintain our life and create and strengthen our immune system. It contributes to the good functioning of the heart and blood vessels.

Problems that can be linked to it include:

- Diseases of the respiratory system.
- Rheumatism (especially in the shoulders).
- Insufficient blood flow.
- Limited respiratory capacity.
- Depression.
- Fatigue.

Postures favoring the optimal function of the lung meridian

1. *Anahatasana*—the puppy dog pose

2. Recommendation: Follow-up with *Marjarasana*—the cat pose, as a neutralization position to create a physical balance after bending back

3. *Bananasana*—the banana position

4. *Bhujangasana*—the cobra pose

5. *Supta Virasana*—the reclined hero pose

6. *Ustrasana*—the camel pose (To harmonize the effort, the counter-position is *Apanasan*—the knees-to-chest pose and rock them right to left)

7. The cat pulling its tail

8. *Savasana*—final meditation, seated.

   Maintain each position for three minutes and 10 minutes *for Savasana*, the final meditation.

The Colon Meridian

This Yang meridian goes from the index finger towards the outside of the arm, up to the shoulder, and then passes along the neck and ends around the nose. It belongs to the Root Chakra.

Proper functioning of this meridian contributes to optimal physical and psychic detoxification. It is imperative to practice letting go to ease the purification. If that meridian is not working optimally, your body produces acidity, which is favorable to the development of many diseases.

Postures favoring the optimal function of the Colon Meridian

1. *Anahatasana*—the puppy dog pose

2. Recommendation: Follow-up with *Marjarasana*—the cat pose as a neutralization position to create a physical balance after bending back

3. *Mandukasana*—the frog pose

4. *Bhujangasana*—the cobra pose

5. *Ustrasana*—the camel pose (To harmonize the effort, the counter-position is *Apanasana*—the knees-to-chest pose and rock them right to left)

6. The cat pulling its tail

7. *Jathara Parivartanasana*—the reclining twist pose

8. *Savasana*—final meditation, seated

Maintain each position for three minutes and 10 minutes for Savasana, the final meditation.

The Stomach Meridian

This Yang meridian starts below the eye in a U shape and heads to the forehead, then passes through the neck, down to the belly, then towards the outside of the leg, and down to the toes. It belongs to the Solar Plexus Chakra. It regulates the stomach and colon functions, and the sexual organs and, for women, the menstrual cycle.

Problems that can be linked to it include:

- Stomach ache.
- Bloating.
- Nauseas.
- Lack of appetite.
- Menstrual pain.

Postures favoring the optimal function
of the Stomach Meridian

1. *Mandukasana*—the frog pose (but with only one leg bent)

2. *Bhujangasana*—the cobra pose

3. *Utthan Pristhasana*—the lizard pose

4. (Recommendation: To create physical harmony, follow-up with *Adho Mukha Svanasana*—downward-facing dog pose)

5. *Janu Sirsasana*—head-to-knee pose. To relax the back, the counter-position is Apanasana—the knees-to-chest pose.

6. *Supta Virasana*—the reclined hero pose

7. *Maksikanagasana*—the dragonfly pose

8. *Jathara Parivartanasana*—the reclining twist pose

9. *Savasana*—seated final meditation to visualize the meridian's proper functioning.

   Maintain each position for three minutes and 10 minutes for Savasana, the final meditation.

The Spleen Meridian

This Yang meridian starts from the big toe towards the interior of the leg, then goes up to the belly and ribs on the exterior of the chest and armpit. It belongs to the earth element and the Solar Plexus Chakra. It is responsible for your digestive system and vital energy. The food you eat is transformed into fuel by this meridian. It also regulates the viscosity of your blood and other body fluids throughout your body.

   Problems that can be linked to it include:

- Digestive problems.
- Thromboses.
- Diabetes.
- Weak states.
- Mood swings.

Postures favoring the optimal function of the Spleen Meridian

1. *Jathara Parivartanasana*—the reclining twist pose.

2. *Mandukasana*—the frog pose.

3. *Utthan Pristhasana*—the lizard pose.

4. (Recommendation: follow-up with *Adho Mukha Svanasana*—downward-facing dog pose to create a physical harmony).

5. *Janu Sirsasana*—head-to-knee pose. To relax the back, the counter-position is the *Apanasana*— the knees-to-chest pose.

6. *Supta Virasana*—the reclined hero pose.

7. *Maksikanagasana*—the dragonfly pose.

8. *Savasana*—seated final meditation to visualize the proper functioning of that meridian.

    Maintain each position for three minutes and 10 minutes for *Savasana*, the final meditation.

The Heart Meridian

This meridian begins around the armpit to go inside the arm and towards the pinky finger. It belongs to the Heart Chakra.

Your heart functions and blood flow are controlled by this meridian. It submits to the influence of your emotions. This is the meridian keeping you alive. In Chinese medicine, it is the origin of your personality.

Problems that can be linked to it include:

- Cardiovascular problems.
- Shoulder and upper-body pain.
- Epilepsy.
- Palpitations.
- States of agitation.

1. Initial meditation to visualize the heart and the color, green.
2. *Bananasana*—the banana position.
3. *Anahatasana*—the puppy dog pose.
4. *Mandukasana*—the frog pose.
5. The cat pulling its tail.
6. *Savasana*—final meditation.

   Maintain each position for three minutes, 5–10 minutes for Savasana.

The Small Intestine Meridian

This Yang meridian starts on the pinky finger's outside and goes towards the back of the arm, then to the shoulder and ear. It belongs to the Solar Plexus Chakra.

Your digestion and metabolism are controlled by this meridian. On the psychic level, it is linked to thoughts and mental capacities.

Problems that can be linked to it include:

- Migraine.
- Dissatisfaction.
- Ear, back, and arm pain.

Postures favoring the optimal function of the Small Intestine Meridian

1. *Nadi Shodana*—alternate nostril breathing exercises
2. *Jathara Parivartanasana*—the reclining twist pose

3. *Mandukasana*—the frog pose

4. *Balasana*—the child's pose

5. *Savasana*—final meditation

Maintain each position for three minutes, 5–10 minutes for *Savasana*.

The Pericardium Meridian

This Yin meridian starts on the outside of the chest, then goes towards the interior of the arm, and down to the middle finger. It belongs to the Heart Chakra.

The pericardium meridian protects the heart and handles blood circulation and the proper functioning of the thyroid gland. On the emotional level, it gives us the capacity to love and maintain deep relationships.

Problems that can be linked to it include:

- Chest pain.
- Vertigo.
- Overstrain.

Postures favoring the optimal function of the Pericardium Meridian

1. Meditation and visualization of the relationships you want

2. *Mandukasana*—the frog pose.

3. *Supta Virasana*—the reclined hero pose.

4. *Ustrasana*—the camel pose.

5. *Bananasana*—the banana position.

6. *Savasana*—final mediation.

Maintain each position for three minutes, 5–10 minutes for Savasana.

The Triple Heater Meridian

This Yang meridian starts behind the ring finger, then goes through the arm up to the shoulder and neck, passes behind the ear, and ends around the eyebrows. It belongs to the Heart Chakra. This triple heater meridian links the other meridians so they can work in a coordinated way. We distinguish three parts: high (the chest), middle (the belly), and low (the pelvic floor).

This meridian eliminates toxins from the body and transforms the food you eat into fuel.

Problems that can be linked to it include:

- Headache.
- Allergies.
- Skin disease.
- Eye and ear diseases.

Postures favoring the optimal function of the Triple Warmer Meridian

1. Meditation and visualization of a body walking in harmony with the outside.
2. *Mandukasana*—the frog pose.
3. *Balasana*—the child's pose.
4. *Jathara Parivartanasana*—the reclining twist pose.
5. *Matsendrasana*—the seated twist pose.
6. *Savasana*—final meditation.

   Maintain each position for three minutes,
   5–10 minutes for *Savasana*.

The Gallbladder Meridian

This Yang meridian starts from outside the eye, then zigzags towards the back of the head, down the neck and chest, and plunges down the leg to end in the toes. It belongs to the Solar Plexus Chakra. It regulates the lymphatic and hormonal systems, as well as the gallbladder. If this meridian functions well, your muscles, tendons, and nails are strong and well built, and you are full of energy. If it is disturbed, you lack tone and vital energy.

Postures favoring the optimal function of the Gallbladder Yang Meridian

1. Initial mediation: slow down the breathing, inhale "positive energy" and exhale "tension"
2. Baddha Konasana—the butterfly
3. Utthan Pristhasana—the dragon
4. Gomukasana—the cow face pose
5. Prapadasana—the tiptoe pose
6. The cat pulling its tail
7. Bhujangasana—the cobra pose
8. Savasana—final meditation

   Maintain each position for three minutes and 5–10 minutes for Savasana, the final meditation.

The Liver Meridian

The Ying liver meridian originates from the big toe, then goes inside the leg and up to the ribs. It belongs to the Solar Plexus Chakra.

If your digestive system and your metabolism work well, that is a sign that Chi flows freely in this meridian. It strengthens your immune system and is responsible for the ideal composition of the blood.

Problems that can be linked to it include:

- Liver disease.
- Chronic issues with the digestive system.
- Colds.
- Pneumonias.
- Addictions.

Postures Favoring the Optimal Function of the Liver Meridian

1. Meditation and creative visualization to live as you want.
2. Baddha Konasana—the butterfly
3. Paschimottanasana—the caterpillar
4. Halasana—the plow pose
5. Jathara Parivartanasana—the reclining twist pose
6. Ananda Balasana—the happy baby pose
7. Viparita Karani—Lying position with legs raised
8. Savasana—final meditation

   Maintain each position for three minutes and 5–10 minutes for Savasana, the final meditation.

8

Yin Yoga Postures

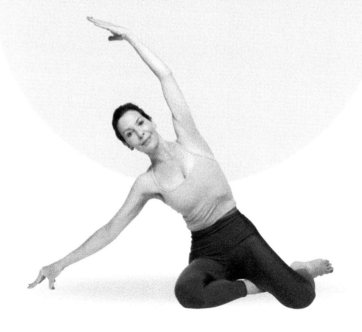

The practice of Yin Yoga helps you connect more with your breathing so you can work on the flexibility of your fasciae, tendons, ligaments, and muscles. The goal is not to go beyond your capabilities. On the contrary, it is to respect your limits and stop well before you reach them to find a comfortable position, which will allow you to keep it for a long time without getting tense. Except where stated, the following poses should be maintained for three to five minutes.

I have illustrated the most appropriate postures with photos to show you how to execute them. It is necessary that you feel right and can relax; that is why we use accessories. Adapt each one to your needs. There might be some you want to execute with no accessory simply because you feel better that way. I have taken photos with accessories to show the postures that most of my students prefer because they find them better. Of course, you can choose an accessory that is not shown in the photo. Rest assured, the written explanations are simple enough to allow you to follow the directions and adapt each position to your own flexibility.

I sometimes recommend using postures to create a balance between two of them, and to relax your muscles before continuing. *Apanasana* is one of those. This posture, with the knees pulled to the chest, relaxes and stretches the lower back. You can rock the knees from right to left to promote muscle extension.

Yin Yoga is a practice that teaches you to accept the present: your body, soul, and spirit, as they are now. Be attentive to your sensations and keep your mind open for continuous adaptation.

It's a good idea to practice Yin Yoga in a calm environment with a comfortable temperature to promote relaxation. Wear clothes that keep you warm and equip yourself with the following accessories, which you can find in any yoga equipment store, or online:

- Two blocks.
- A belt.
- A blanket.
- A bolster.

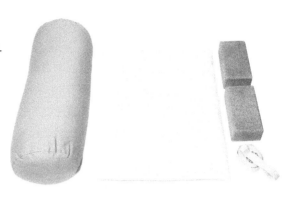

1. Anahatasana - The Puppy Dog Pose

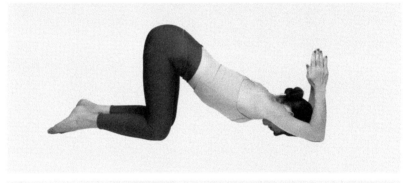

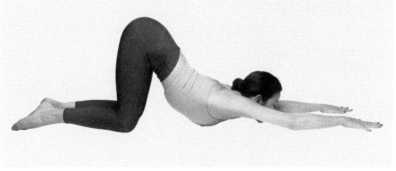

The benefits of this posture

This posture gives flexibility to your upper and middle back and shoulders. It stimulates your heart and improves posture.

The muscles used are the spinal erectors (erector spinae), the trapezium (trapezius), the shoulder girdle, and the diaphragm.

You can use *Anahatasana* to prepare your body to bend backwards for the bridge or the camel pose, and as a position to open your posture and the heart.

How to reproduce this posture

Get on all fours. Bring your hands forward until you can rest your chest on the floor. Keep your hips and knees vertically aligned; look for the stretching sensation in the back of the coccyx to promote the stretching of the lower back. Keep your hands aligned with your shoulders.

Alternatives and modifications

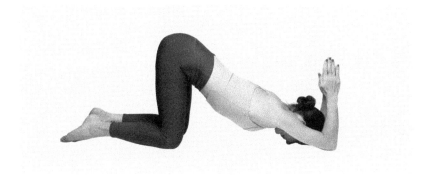

If you feel pain or tingling in your hands or fingers when you lift your arms, you can spread your forearms further and position the bolster under your belly or below your elbows. If that is not comfortable for your knees, place a blanket beneath them.

In the case of shoulder problems, you can rest only on one elbow, and rest the head on the other one.

2. Ankle stretch

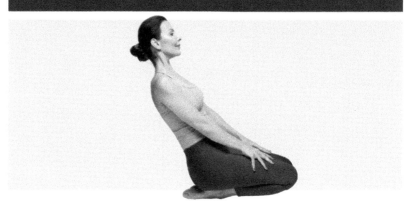

The benefits of this posture

The stretching of your ankles brings greater strength and flexibility to that joint. This posture is recommended to maintain squats on your toes (shown later in this chapter).

How to reproduce this posture

Begin by sitting on your heels. You can place the blanket beneath your knees to reduce the pressure. If joint pain in your knees and ankles persists, avoid this position.

Alternatives and modifications

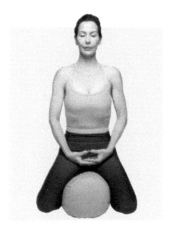

If you feel pain other than stretching in the knees or ankles (in the back, hips, etc.), you can place a cushion or multiple blankets beneath your knees to make the position more comfortable. If you suffer from knee problems, I recommend you fold a blanket multiple times and place it between your knees and thighs.

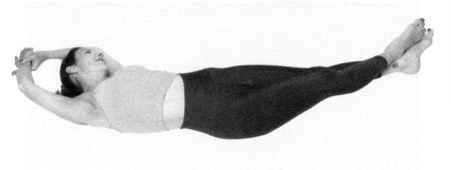

The benefits of this posture

Bananasana is an extraordinary stretch for the obliques, so you benefit from relaxation along all the sides of the body. This improves the spine's mobility in lateral flexion by lengthening the iliotibial band at the top of the lateral rib cage.

How to reproduce this posture

Lie on the ground with legs extended, stretch the arms above the head, and cross the fingers. Bring the arms and the legs towards the right, while keeping the hips and buttocks in the center. Maintain the position until you feel your muscles relax Then you can go further to the right and intensify the stretching. Then do it on the other side.

Alternatives and modifications

If you have tingling or an unpleasant feeling in your raised arms, you can put a blanket under them, or place them on your stomach. If you have lower back problems (including a hernia or sciatica), focus on stretching your back, not the angle. You can place a cushion under your knees to be more comfortable.

4. Baddha Konasana - The Butterfly

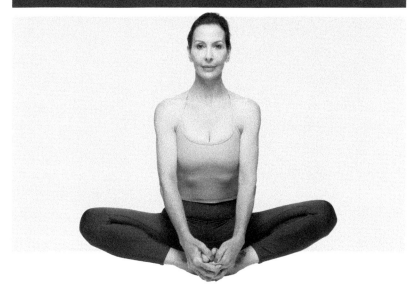

The benefits of this posture

The Butterfly allows the stretching of your lower back and improves your mobility by reducing the impact on the back of your legs. By keeping your feet close to the pubis, the effects of this position can be reduced. The adductors (adductor longus, brevis, magnus, minimus, pectineus and gracilis) are stretched. However, if your feet are far from the pubis, the seat bones are involved and elongated.

How to reproduce this posture

Sit on a folded blanket. Then join the soles of your feet and bring them closer to your pubis. Allow your back to stretch and bend your body forward, while holding your feet to bring your head closer to them. If possible, use your elbows to push down on your knees to intensify the effects of the posture.

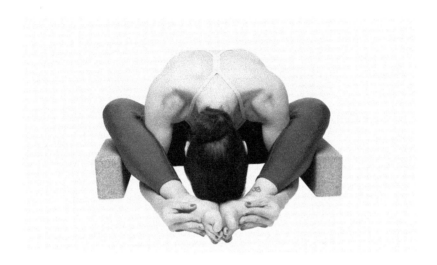

To make the position more comfortable and allow you to relax more, place a block under each thigh and put your feet further from your pubis. This way, your neck can relax, and you can fully let go simply by focusing on your breathing.

If your knees do not like this position, or you just had surgery to the meniscus, ACL or PCL, look at the next position, *Janu Sirsasana*.

If you suffer from sciatica, lift your hips by sitting on the blocks or bolster so your knees are lower than your hips.

In the case of a lumbar hernia, practice *Baddha Konasana* while keeping your back straight and well stretched.

5. Janu Sirsasana - Head-to-Knee Pose

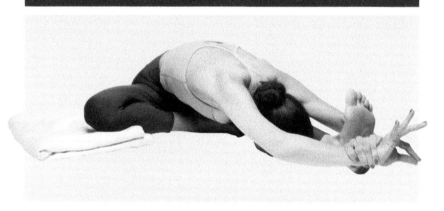

The benefits of this posture

This posture allows you to stretch the backs of your legs, one after the other, while protecting the bent knee. You can place a folded blanket, or a block, under that knee so it can rest without tension. The seat bones (semimembranosus, semitendinosus, and biceps femoris) lengthen.

You stimulate and promote your digestive system's functioning with the torso bending towards the thigh.

How to reproduce this posture

Sit on your mat with your legs stretched. First, bend the right knee and bring the foot against the opposite thigh.

Alternatives and modifications

If you have just had surgery for the meniscus or the cruciate ligaments, place the block or the blanket under your knees, so they can fully relax without constraint. Wait five to six weeks after the surgery, and with the approval of your doctor before doing this posture.

6. Supta Baddha Konasana
The Reclined Butterfly

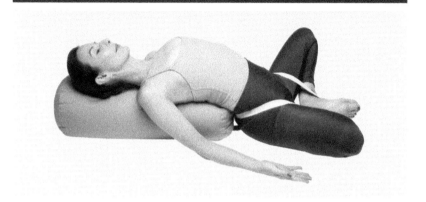

The benefits of this posture

This posture opens and gives flexibility to the hips. It stretches your adductors (adductor longus, magnus, brevis, minimus, gracilis, and pectineus).

If you suffer from a hernia or sciatica, this is an extraordinary alternative to *Baddha Konasana* (bent forward), because you create space between vertebrae thanks to the light lumbar curvature, which allows the vertebral liquid to be absorbed.

How to reproduce this posture

Sit and place the soles of your feet together close to the pubis. Put a belt around your waist and feet, then tighten it until you feel your hip opening deepen. Then you can lie on the bolster previously placed behind you. Your lumbar vertebrae and the rest of the spine will rest on the cushion.

Alternatives and modifications

If your knees do not touch the ground, place a block beneath each knee for support; this will allow them to flex more, and the position will be more comfortable.

If you have kyphosis, and your neck is not resting on the bolster, place another cushion under your head.

7. The Cat Pulling its Tail posture

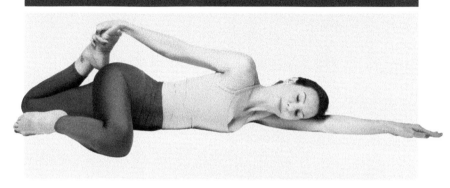

The benefits of this posture

This posture allows you to stretch the quadriceps (*vastus medialis, vastus lateralis, vastus intermedius,* and *rectus femoris*). This posture is more accessible than the reclined hero pose and allows you to work deeply and gently.

How to reproduce this posture

Lie on your right side and rest your head on your right arm. Keep the right leg stretched and bend the left knee to 90°. Catch and hold the right heel and pull it gently towards your buttocks with your left hand. Aim to push the heel away to intensify the stretch and keep your pelvis neutral, and push the coccyx in. The lower back tends to hollow out, which reduces the stretching effect. If the position is no longer effective physiologically, tilt the pelvis and place it back in a neutral position, meaning that you align both the iliac crests and pubis.

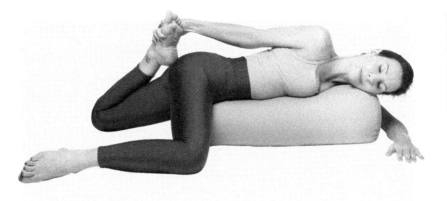

If you want to make this posture more accessible and more comfortable for your back, take a bolster and lie over it. Your head and pubis are then supported. This version will allow you to maintain the pelvis in a physiologically more correct, more neutral position, and will intensify the feeling of stretching.

8. *Paschimottanasana* - The Caterpillar

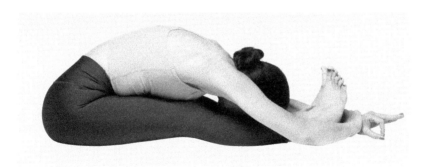

The benefits of this posture

This posture allows the stretching of your legs (*semimembrasosus, semitendinosus, biceps femoris*) and lower back (*quadratus lumborum*).

The compression strengthens the digestive organs and promotes the elimination of toxins.

How to reproduce this posture

To ensure your pelvis tilts forward, I suggest you take a blanket, fold it over many times, and place it under your seat bones to promote a tilt. Then stretch your legs forward.

Alternatives and modifications

If the flexibility of your posterior chain does not allow you to bend forward:

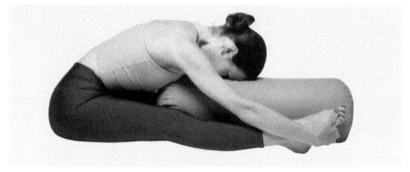

A)   Place a bolster on your thighs, then bend over it.

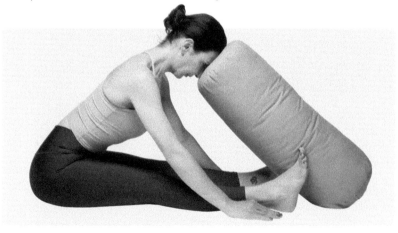

B) Place the bolster diagonally to rest your forehead on it. You can hold it with your feet to be more stable and let go more.

In the case of sciatica, place a block, a cushion or a blanket under your seat bones, so your hips are higher than your knees.

If you have a lumbar hernia, it is preferable not to do this posture.

9. *Balasana* - The Child's Pose

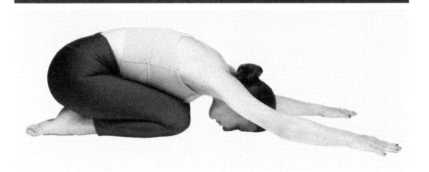

The benefits of this posture

This posture allows you to relax your lower back *(quadratus lumborum)* and your pelvis. It will lead you into a relaxed state and interior peace.

Your forehead (third eye, the Ajna Chakra) resting on the ground stimulates your intuition.

How to reproduce this posture

Sit on your heels. Your knees can be slightly apart or together, depending on how you feel. If you are pregnant, you need to keep them apart for greater comfort. Bend over your thighs and stretch your hands forward to fully take advantage of the stretching of your spine.

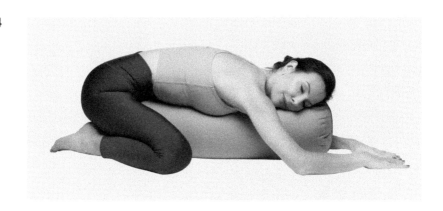

Alternatives and modifications

To be even more comfortable, and if you suffer from knee pain, you can place a bolster between your knees and lie over it. Close your eyes and practice letting go.

10. *Uttanasana* - Standing Forward Fold

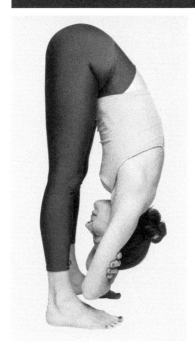

The benefits of this posture

This posture will help you loosen up your posterior chain, especially your hamstrings *(semimembranosus, semitendinosus,* and *biceps femoris)* and your lower back *(quadratus lumborum).* Your digestive system will be stimulated, and the posture will lead you into introspection, because you are folded onto yourself.

How to reproduce this posture

Stand with your feet aligned with your shoulders. You can bend forward, knees slightly bent, and hang your arms or grab the opposite elbow to further lengthen your spine. Deepen your breath and aim to gently tense the knees.

Alternatives and modifications

If you suffer from sciatica, keep your knees bent.
In the case of a lumbar hernia, it is preferable not to do this posture.

11. *Utthan Pristhasana* - The Lizard Pose

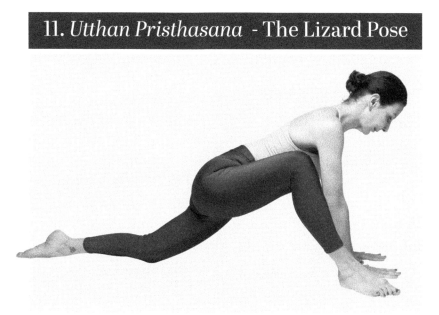

The benefits of this posture

Thanks to this posture, tension in the hip flexors, including the psoas and the quadriceps *(vastus medialis, vastus lateralis, vastus intermedius, rectus femoris)* will be reduced, and you will notice a feeling of relaxation in the hip joint.

How to reproduce this posture

Get on all fours. First, place the right foot next to your hands, then push back the opposite knee. Then, gently push your pelvis forward to feel the stretching in the hip flexors.

Alternatives and modifications

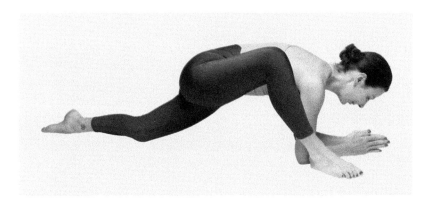

If you feel some tension behind the knee, place a blanket beneath it.

If you want to go further in this posture, and have the flexibility for it, lower the forearms to the ground. To open your hip even more, raise the interior of your forward foot to promote an external rotation of the knee. You can also place the arm inside the foot and slightly push the calf to open more.

12. *Mandukasana* - The Frog Pose

The benefits of this posture

By practicing the frog pose, you stretch the adductors *(adductor longus, adductor brevis, adductor magnus, adductor minimus, gracilis,* and *pectineus)*. The adductor muscles are frequently used in lateral movements. This posture improves their flexibility and facilitates those movements.

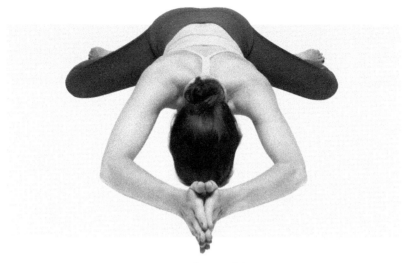

How to reproduce this posture

Begin by placing yourself in the child's pose, then bring the arms forward, and spread your knees. If you want to go further, spread your feet to have them on the same line as your knees, and push your hips backward to stretch more.

Alternatives and modifications

For greater comfort, you can place the bolster between your legs and lay your upper body on top of it. If you have shoulder problems, I suggest you keep the arms apart instead of pulling them forward.

13. *Ananda Balasana*
The Happy Baby Pose

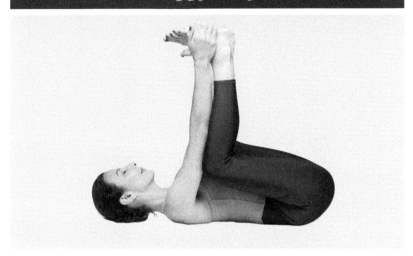

The benefits of this posture

This posture relaxes and masses your sacroiliac joint, as well as your lumbar vertebrae. An opening of the hips allows you to determine its intensity by using the strength of your arms.

The digestive system is stimulated because your thighs are near the center of your body.

How to reproduce this posture

Lie on your back, knees close to your chest. Catch the soles of your feet, your ankles, or the back of your legs. Bring your feet towards you to align them with your knees and aim to bring the knees closer to the ground. Make sure your trapezes and shoulders remain relaxed and far from your ears.

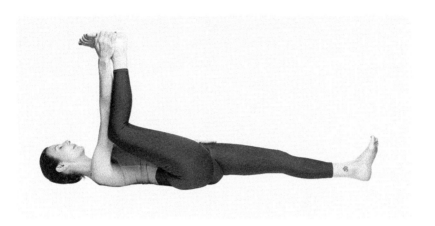

Alternatives and modifications

If the backs of your legs are tense, you can place a belt around your feet to bring them closer to your chest more easily. It is important for the coccyx to remain on the ground.

Another modification is to take only one leg at a time.

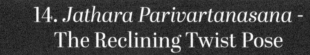

14. *Jathara Parivartanasana -* The Reclining Twist Pose

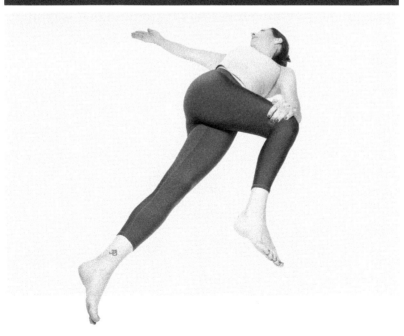

The benefits of this posture

This posture will relax your spine and promote relaxation. It improves and supports the flexibility in torsion and stretches the hips, the *gluteus medius* and the *piriformis*.

How to reproduce this posture

Lie on your back, stretch your left leg, and pull the right knee towards your chest. Maintain the position to reduce tension in your lower back *(quadratus lumborum)* and hip flexor, the *iliopsoas*. Then, turn on your left side and look the other way. Try to keep your shoulder girdle on the ground and apply a light pressure with the left hand on the right knee to push it down.

Alternatives and modifications

If your bent knee or shoulders do not touch the ground, place a block or a belt beneath those zones to promote relaxation.

It is possible to do that torsion with both legs; all you need to do is to bend the leg that was extended. That way, both will be oriented towards the left (one on top of the other), with your eyes looking the other way. That intensifies the stretching.

15. *Supta Virasana* - The Reclined Hero Pose

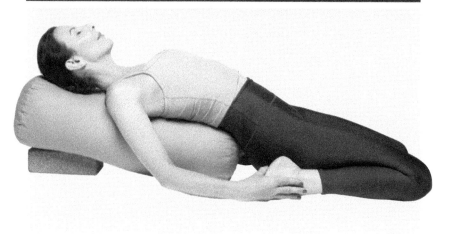

The benefits of this posture

This posture allows you to open and deeply extend the sacroiliac joint. It stretches the hip *flexors (iliopsoas, sartorius, tensor fasciae latae)* and the quadriceps *(vastus medialis, vastus lateralis, vastus intermedius,* and *rectus femoris).* If you can keep your heels outside your hips, you will benefit from an internal rotation of that joint, unlike the external rotations that are practiced way too often.

How to reproduce this posture

Sit on your heels, with knees together and heels outside your buttocks. If you have unpleasant tension in the ankles, place a blanket beneath them. First, go backward with the upper body. You can place your hands on the ground to hold you. If you want to go further, rest your elbows on the ground or lie down completely.

Alternatives and modifications

I suggest you use a bolster under your back to make this posture more comfortable and allow yourself to focus on letting go completely. If necessary, place blocks under the bolster to make the *Supta Virasana* even more accessible and to raise the upper body a little more.

In the case of strained knees, I suggest the half-saddle, which means placing one leg, with a bent knee, foot on the ground towards the buttock, and the other one in the initial position of the reclined hero pose, then go backward with the upper body.

16. *Gomukasana* - The Cow Face Pose

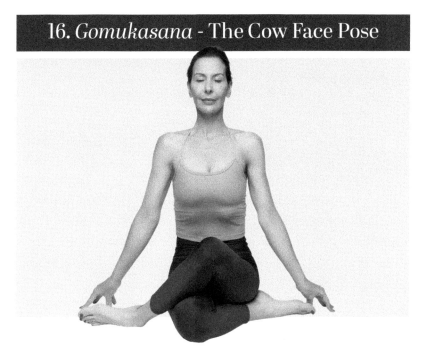

The benefits of this posture

This position allows you to open and relax your hips. By practicing it, you contribute to balancing the internal and external rotations of your knees to create harmony and optimal functioning of that joint.

Get on all fours. Cross the right knee over the left knee as high as possible. Then, you can sit, making sure that both seat bones are on the ground. Open the knees and stay in this position.

Do you want to go further? Lift your arms and bring the right arm under the other, cross the elbows to catch the wrists or, if possible, place your hands in the prayer position.

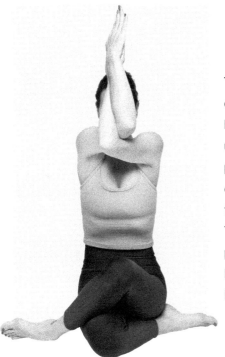

Alternatives and modifications

To allow your hips to relax and your pelvis to move in a better way, place a blanket under your seat bones to promote an anteversion. You can bend forward to benefit from a lower back stretching. To help you in this position, place a bolster under your belly or forehead and rest on it.

17. Halasana - The Plow Pose

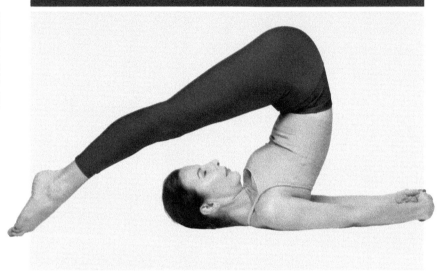

The benefits of this posture

This posture stretches and lengthens the spine. It also improves the blood circulation in your head and brain, thanks to the inverted gravity. *Halasana* massages compressed internal organs. The high pressure stimulates their working. Because the organs go up, you reduce the intra-abdominal pressure and weight on the pelvic floor. Your lungs are drained.

I strongly suggest that you practice this posture to reduce anxiety and stress and bring yourself into a calmed and rested state.

How to reproduce this posture

Lie on the ground. Lift your hips and hold your back with your hands. Hold the body's weight on the shoulder girdle rather than on the neck. If it is painful, avoid bringing the legs too close to the ground. You can place your legs on a bolster. If you want to relax and open your shoulders and trapeze more, cross your fingers behind your back and create a maximum of distance between ears and shoulders.

Alternatives and modifications

To make this position more comfortable, place a blanket under the neck and shoulders.

You do not feel ready for such an inversion? Lie on the ground, legs stretched against a wall, and place a bolster under your buttock to benefit from a modified inverted position and allow yourself to take advantage of those benefits.

If you suffer from high blood pressure, I suggest you practice the previous position, because you absolutely need to avoid having your head below your hips.

If you suffer from glaucoma, avoid this posture.

18. *Karnapidasana* - The Ear Pressure Pose

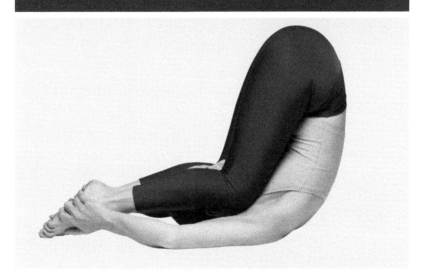

The benefits of this posture

This posture stretches and lengthens your spine. It improves blood circulation. It also improves the blood circulation in the head and brain, thanks to the inverted gravity. *Karnapidasana* massages your compressed internal organs. The thigh pressure stimulates their working. In addition, you reduce the intra-abdominal pressure because the organs go up and the weight on the pelvic floor disappears. Your lungs are drained.

I strongly suggest that you practice this posture to reduce anxiety and stress, and to bring yourself into a calmed and rested state.

How to reproduce this posture

Lie on the ground. Lift your hips and bring your legs behind your head, bend your knees, and place your hands on your feet. Bring your knees towards the ground.

Hold the body's weight on the shoulder girdle rather than on the neck. If it is painful, avoid bringing the legs or knees too close to the ground.

If you wish to relax and open your shoulders and trapeze more, cross your fingers behind your back and create a maximum distance between your ears and shoulders.

Alternatives and modifications

To make this position more comfortable, place a blanket under your neck and shoulders.

If you do not feel ready for such in inversion? Lie on the ground, legs stretched against a wall, and place a bolster under your buttocks to benefit from a modified inverted position and allow yourself to take advantage of those benefits.

If you suffer from high blood pressure, I suggest you practice the *Halasana*, because you absolutely need to avoid having your head below your hips.

If you suffer from glaucoma, avoid this posture.

In the case of a cervical disc hernia, please refrain from practicing this posture.

19. *Supta Padangustasana* A, B, & C - Stretching the Hamstrings

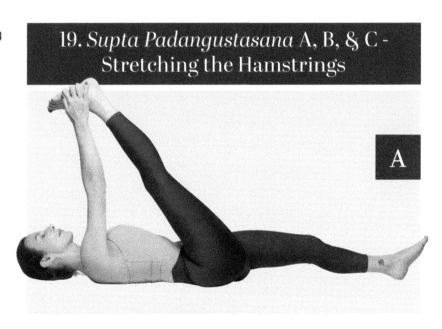

The benefits of this posture

This posture allows you to stretch the back of your legs *(semimembranosus, semitendinosus, biceps femoris)* and the *psoas* of the leg, which remains stretched on the ground.

If you have a teacher or a therapist practicing with you, by placing their foot or their hand on the *psoas*, they can stretch it in an efficient and intense manner.

How to reproduce this posture

A) Lie on the ground. Lift the right leg and bend it, then stretch gently as much as you can. Catch the ankle or the knee and gently bring the leg towards you. If necessary, take a belt and place it around the foot to hold it. Take advantage of this elongation without lifting or tensing your shoulders and trapezius.

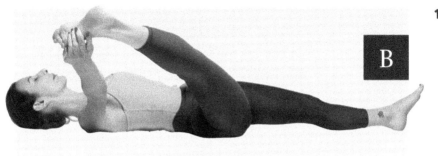

B) Bring the right leg towards the right and keep it elongated. Aim to keep the shoulder girdle and the hips on the ground.

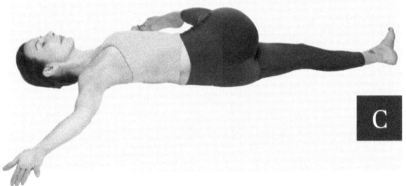

C) Cross the right leg to the opposite side and keep it elongated. Make sure you do not raise the right hip, stay rooted and stabilize the pelvis. Do the same thing on the left side.

Alternatives and modifications

To make the posture easier, you can bend the leg that stays on the ground, knowing this facilitates the elongation of the back of the leg, but you will no longer benefit from the relaxation of the *psoas*/hip flexors.

Use a belt to hold your feet. In the case of a very flexible sacroiliac joint, only do *Supta Padangustasana* A & B, and avoid twisting.

In the case of a hernia, practice only *Supta Padangustasana* A and make sure your lower back remains neutral.

20. *Bhujangasana* - The Cobra Pose

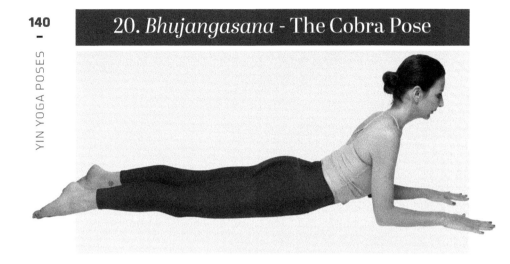

The benefits of this posture

This posture stretches the right abdomen muscle, the rectus abdominis. An improvement of the posture thanks to the chest opening, and correction in the case of kyphosis. Toning and strengthening of the posterior muscles, such as the square muscle of the loins, the quadratus lumborum and the erector spinae.

Bhujangasana is highly recommended in cases of lumbar hernia and sciatica.

How to Reproduce this Posture

Lie on your stomach. Place the forearms on the ground to allow you to raise your chest. Keep your shoulders far from your ears and get your head out of the trapeze. Relax your buttocks and lower back. Maintain this position.

If you are pregnant, it is preferable not to do this posture and replace it with *Marjarasana*—The Cat Pose.

21. *Urdhva Mukha Svanasana* - The Upward Facing Dog Pose

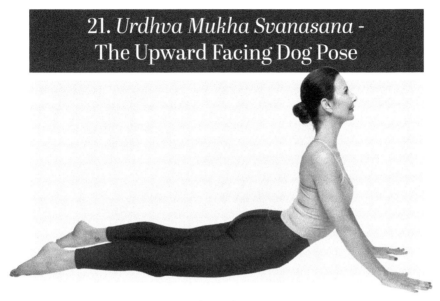

The benefits of this posture

The stretching of the right abdomen muscle, the *rectus abdominis*. An improvement of the posture thanks to the chest opening, and correction in the case of kyphosis. Toning and strengthening of the posterior muscles, such as the square muscle of the loins, the *quadratus lumborum* and the *erector spinae*.

Urdhva Mukha Svanasana is highly recommended in cases of lumbar hernia and sciatica.

How to reproduce this posture

Place your hands below your shoulders and, with a deep breath, extend the arms to move yourself up to the dog position, with your head high. Shoulders remain distant from your ears. Keep pulling your shoulders back to promote postural opening.

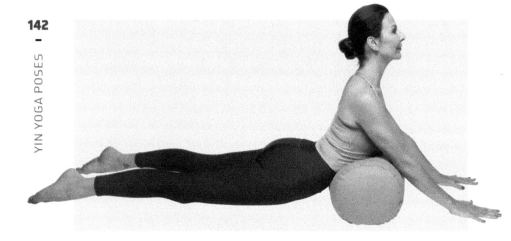

Alternatives and modifications

Place the bolster under your belly or ribs, for better support in the posture and to promote concentration and breathing. You can spread your legs if you feel a tension in your lower back. To remove pressure on the pubis, place a blanket, folded at your convenience, under that zone.

If you are pregnant, don't do this posture; replace it with *Marjarasana*—The Cat Pose.

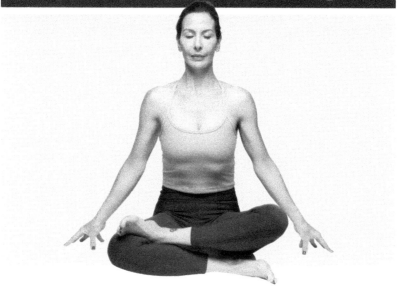

The benefits of this posture

This posture opens the hips in external rotation. Additionally, it adds flexibility to the buttocks (*gluteus medius and gluteus minimus*), the iliotibial band, and the tensor fascia muscle. *Agnistambhasana* is highly recommended for people with the iliotibial band syndrome[2].

How to reproduce this posture

Begin by sitting cross-legged. Place your tibias parallel to the front of the mat. Place a leg on top of the other and maintain this alignment. Keep your feet bent to protect your knees. To stretch more, bend forward with arms stretched and fingers on the ground.

---

2   The *ilio-tibial* band syndrome, or *ilio-tibial* tract syndrome (ITTS), also called the "windshield wiper syndrome," or "tendinitis of the tensor muscle of the *fascia lata*," is a type of tendinitis of the knee.

Alternatives and modifications

If your knees do not touch the ground, or hurt you, place a blanket or a block beneath them. If that posture is unpleasant, try it with only one leg bent and the other elongated. Then switch. To promote the tilt of the pelvis, place a cushion under your seat bones.

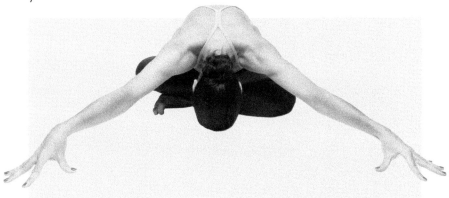

23. *Malasana* - The Garland Pose

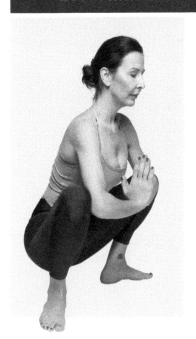

The benefits of this posture

This posture gives flexibility to your hips, the insides of your thighs and your adductors *(adductor longus, brevis, magnus, minimus, pectineus,* and *gracilis). Malasana* strengthens your ankles and relaxes your lower back.

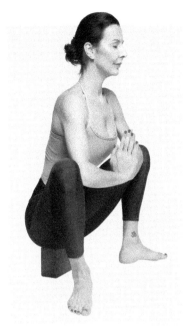

How to reproduce this posture

Start in the standing position, with your legs aligned with your hips. Squat and bring your arms forward, hands in prayer position. Use your elbows to press lightly against the insides of your knees to push them further apart.

Alternatives and modifications

If your heels do not touch the ground, you can fold a blanket and place it beneath them. You can use a block or two to sit on; the position becomes then more meditative.

24. *Prapadasana* - The Tiptoe Pose

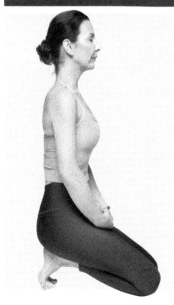

The benefits of this posture

This posture strengthens your ankles and feet, and tones your quadriceps (*vastus lateralis, vastus medialis, vastus intermedius, rectus femoris*).

How to reproduce this posture

Place yourself in a standing position, legs together. Start by putting yourself in demi-pointes, with your heels lifted and fix a point for better balance. Slowly bend your knees to descend into the tiptoe pose, then drop your knees to the floor.

Alternatives and modifications

If it is difficult to maintain this position, why not place a blanket or a block beneath your heels to stabilize them?

25. Ustrasana - The Camel Pose

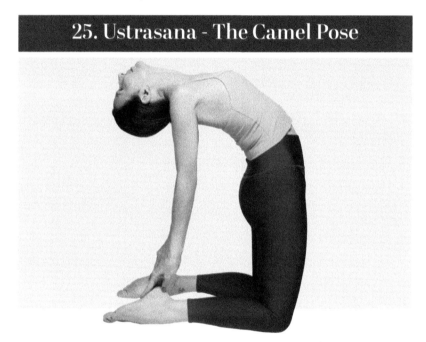

The benefits of this posture

You open your posture and shoulders to tone your back *(quadratus lumborum)*. You benefit from a stretch of the large rectus abdominis muscle.

Ustrasana is recommended if you have a lumbar hernia.

Get on your knees, slightly apart. Lift your arms and stretch your back, then bend backward. You can place your hands on your buttocks, or if you want to go further, point the toes and put your hands on your heels. Maintain the position, making sure your buttocks stay relaxed. If you feel your muscles relax, you can place your feet flat (as in the picture).

Alternatives and modifications

If your neck is too tense, keep your toes aligned with your arms and control the tension with your body. You can also keep looking straight ahead to avoid neck tension and thus protect it.

Place blocks vertically beside your feet to place your hands on. To protect your knees, place a blanket beneath them.

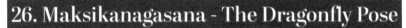

26. Maksikanagasana - The Dragonfly Pose

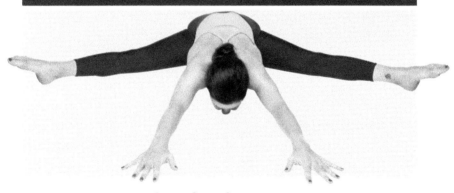

The benefits of this posture

This posture opens the hips and gives them flexibility. You stretch the adductors (adductor longus, magnus, brevis, minimus, pectineus and gracilis) as well as the backs of your legs (semimembranosus, semitendinosus, and biceps femoris).

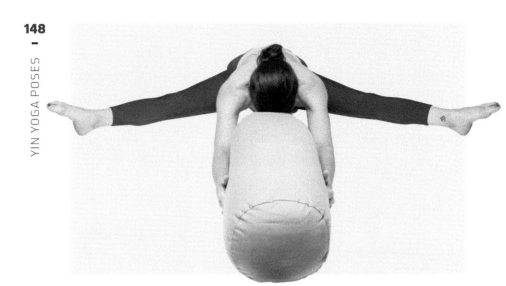

How to reproduce this posture

Sit on the mat and place a folded blanket beneath your seat bones to promote the tilt of your pelvis. Start by slowly spreading your legs, making sure your knees do not turn outwards. Do not force it; find a position that allows you to breathe deeply and let go. You can always open more after a few minutes.

Alternatives and modifications

To promote the tilt of the pelvis, place your hands behind your hips and press on them to move your body weight forward and maintain the position.

Place a bolster on the ground, lengthwise, and place the belly on top of it. This stimulates the digestive system.

If you prefer, place the bolster upright, diagonally, and place your forehead on it to change the position. This stimulates the third eye. Focus on your back, so it stays straight and elongated, and the pelvis stays in anteversion.

27. Adho Mukha Svanasana
The Downward-facing Dog Pose

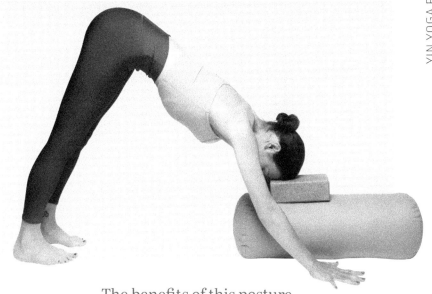

The benefits of this posture

This posture stretches the backs of the legs and the lumbar vertebrae; it can serve as a preparation for other, more advanced, inversions. The downward-facing dog pose acts as corrective for scoliosis and helps realign the spine. You can use it to create a balance inside your body, after forward- or backward-bending postures.

How to reproduce this posture

Place yourself on all fours with your shoulders, hips, and knees aligned. Inhale and extend your legs backward, lower the heels towards the ground to stretch your posterior chain, including the backs of your legs (semimembranosus, semitendinosus, biceps femoris, and gluteus maximus) and calves (gastrocnemius and soleus).

Alternatives and modifications to this posture

To promote a relaxed state, place the bolster upright on the ground and place your head on top of it. If your head does not reach it, place a block on top of it to rest your forehead.

28. Rajakapotasana - The Pigeon

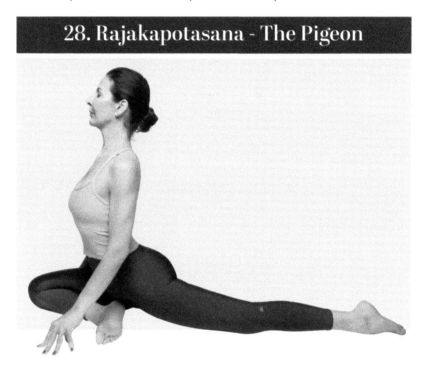

The benefits of this posture

This posture stretches the hips in external rotation and improves their mobility. In addition, it gives flexibility to the psoas and the lateral muscles of the hip, such as the *gluteus medius* and the *piriformis*, which relieves piriformis syndrome. The loin square, the *quadratus lumborum*, is toned up, lifting the upper body. Blood circulation in the area is stimulated, and you benefit from a large pelvis amplitude.

How to reproduce this posture

Put yourself in the downward-facing dog pose. Then bring the right foot behind the left hand and place the knee forward. If you have no tension in the knee, push your tibia forward towards the ground while opening the angle of your knee a little and extend the back leg. Make sure your hips stay parallel.

Alternatives and modifications

Place a blanket or a block under your hip on the side of the bent knee to keep the pelvis aligned. You can lie forward. Keep the forward foot bent to protect the knee.

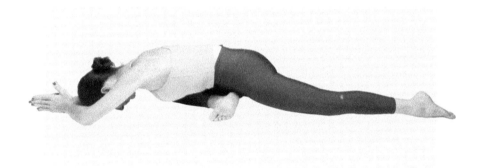

29. Supta Kapotasana - The Reclined Pigeon Pose, Variation to Stretch the Piriformis

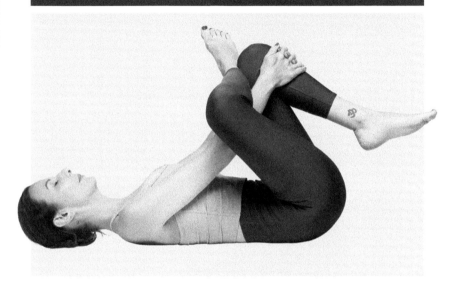

The benefits of this posture

This posture stretches the hips and relieves the piriformis syndrome. The reclined pigeon pose is accessible to everyone and promotes the relaxation of the sacroiliac joint.

How to reproduce this posture

Lie on your mat and lift your legs. Cross the right leg over the left and pass your hands between your thighs to catch your left tibia. Direct your attention to keeping the bent knee distanced from the center to intensify the stretching. Keep the shoulders far from the ears and maintain slow, deep breathing.

I suggest you bend the foot to protect the bent knee. Make sure the coccyx remains on the ground. If your lower back is tense or painful, place a folded blanket under your buttocks to raise yourself a little.

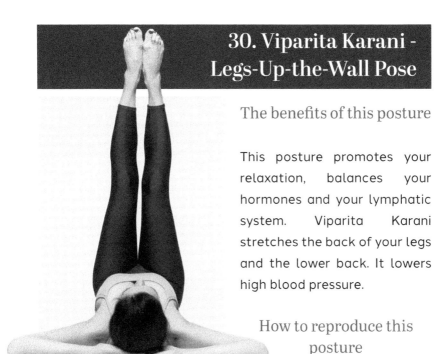

30. Viparita Karani - Legs-Up-the-Wall Pose

The benefits of this posture

This posture promotes your relaxation, balances your hormones and your lymphatic system. Viparita Karani stretches the back of your legs and the lower back. It lowers high blood pressure.

How to reproduce this posture

Sit with a hip next to a wall and bent knees resting on the ground. Lay on your back and bring your extended legs against the wall to create a 90° angle between your legs and chest. Thanks to the wall, you can hold the extended legs without effort and fully fight water retention. You can let go and focus on your breathing.

Alternatives and modifications

You can change your arm positions to promote the opening of your chest. Place them on your sides, aligned with your shoulders.

To relax your lower back even more, you can place a blanket or a block under your lumbar vertebrae. Lifting the pelvis reduces tension and pain in that region. In addition, you reduce the intra-abdominal pressure on the pelvic floor, which lifts the organs and prevents incontinence and organ descent.

I strongly recommend this posture in the postnatal phase and during the premenopausal and menopausal stages.

31. Marjarasana - The Cat Pose

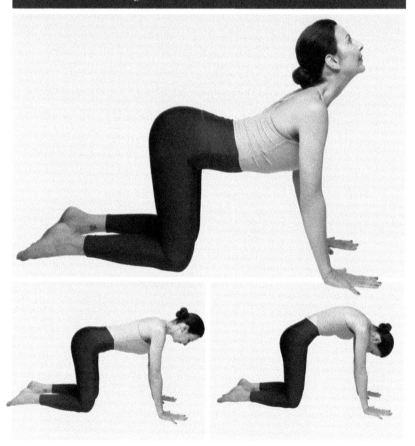

The benefits of this posture

This posture relaxes the upper-back muscles, including the trapeze and rhomboid, as well as the shoulders. You extend and lengthen the back extensors, erector spinae and the multifidus. I recommend that you integrate Marjarasana between Yin Yoga postures to harmonize your effort and stimulate your blood circulation.

How to reproduce this posture

Inhale and lower the lower back while looking up. Exhale, round your back, and direct your gaze towards your navel to help lengthen and round your back.

Repeat this posture four times.

Alternatives and modifications

To involve the pelvic floor muscle more, and to ensure a hip-knee vertical alignment, I suggest you squeeze a cushion between your thighs.

32. Padmasana - The Lotus Pose

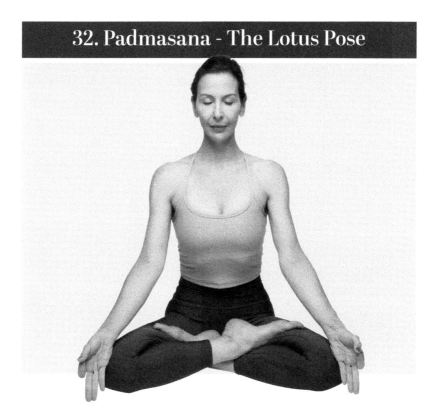

The benefits of this posture

This position allows you to improve your posture. Thanks to the crossed legs, your back is perfectly extended. You also remove spine tension and reduce intra-abdominal pressure.

How to reproduce this posture

Sit with your back straight. You can place a folded blanket beneath your seat bones to facilitate their tilt. Next, cross the right leg over the groin and then place the left leg on top.

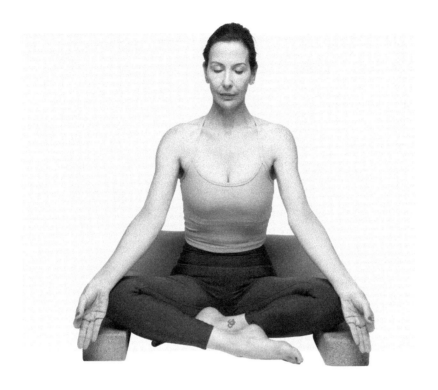

Alternatives and modifications

To facilitate the lotus position, you can cross only the right leg over the groin and fold the other one normally on the ground. By placing a block under each knee, you can remove the tension and give more support to your knees. If that does not suit you, simply cross your legs.

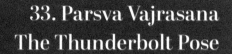

33. Parsva Vajrasana
The Thunderbolt Pose

The benefits of this posture

This posture extends the intercostal muscles and creates space between your ribs. You will also benefit from lengthening your obliques. Finally, you strengthen the stability of your shoulder girdle and pelvic floor.

Parsva Vajrasana can help correct scolioses.

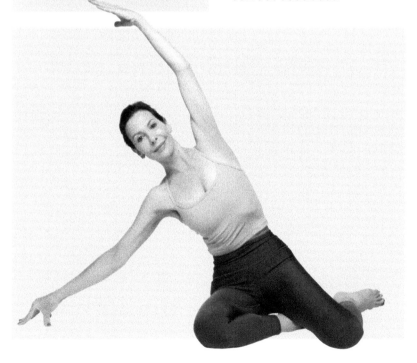

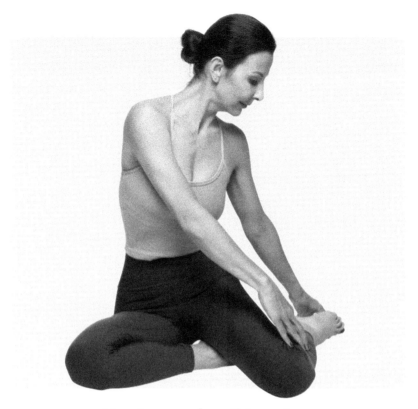

How to reproduce this posture

Begin by sitting on your knees, then slide over to your right side.
Stretch the left arm over your ears and extend it. Make sure your
shoulders stay far from your ears.

Same thing to the left.

The Thunderbolt Pose with Rotation

Keep your arms towards the ground and bring the left arm to
the outside of your right knee to promote rotation. Keep the
spine extended and then turn yourself to maintain the maximum
space between your vertebrae.

Same thing to the left.

In the case of a lumbar hernia or sciatica, do not do this posture.

34. Salabhasana - The Grasshopper Pose

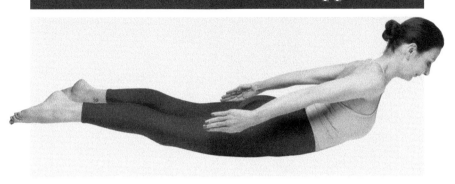

The benefits of this posture

This posture strengthens the posterior chain, including the back of the legs *(semimembranosus, semitendinosus, bicep femoris)*, the buttocks *(gluteus maxiumus* and *minimus)*, the square muscle of the loins *(quadratus lumborum)*, and the abdominal-lumbar belt. Opening this posture improves your pulmonary capacity.

You can use this position to prepare your body before your Yin Yoga session, or during it, to harmonize and balance your practice.

How to reproduce this posture

Lie on your stomach with your arms along your body. While inhaling, lift your legs and arms. Make sure your neck stays aligned with the rest of your spine. You can imagine a tennis ball between your chin and chest to facilitate an optimal neck position.

Alternatives and modifications

If you are pregnant, you can replace Salabhasana with Marjarasana—The Cat Pose.

Salabhasana is highly recommended for a discal hernia.

35. Matsyendrasana - The Seated Twist Pose

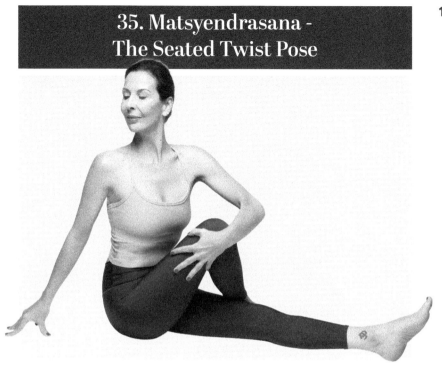

The benefits of this posture

This posture strengthens the back extensors (erector spinae) and the transverse muscles *(transversus abdominus)*, the deepest abdominal layer. Matsyendrasana stimulates and massages the digestive system. This seated twist pose can help correct scolioses and maintain a toned and flexible spine.

How to reproduce this posture

Sit with legs extended. Cross the right leg over the left and place your foot firmly on the ground. Then, lift your arms and extend your back, maintaining the seat bones on the ground. Catch the right knee with your left arm. Inhale to extend your back, and exhale to return to intensify the torsion.

Same thing on the left.

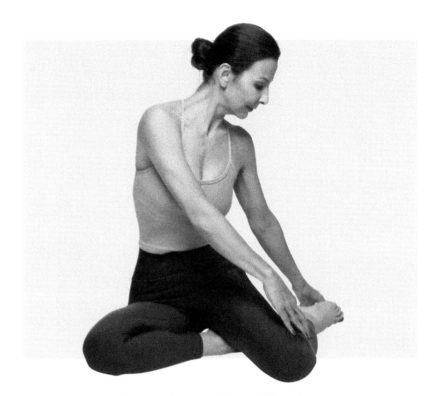

Alternatives and modifications

If crossing one leg over the other is unpleasant for your knees, maintain the leg inside your thigh.

To intensify this position, you can bend your left leg, then cross the right leg over it. Then, bring your left arm inside the right leg, and bring that knee closer to your chest. Place your right arm behind your back and catch your left wrist, if you are flexible enough.

36. Navasana - The Boat Pose

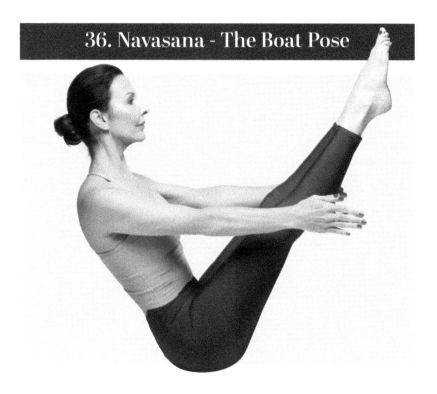

The benefits of this posture

This posture strengthens the abdominal-lumbar belt, including the square of the loins *(quadratus lumborum)*, the transverse muscles *(transversus abdominus)*, and hip flexors *(iliopsoas)*.

I suggest you use this posture to prepare your body for Yin Yoga practice, or integrate it to harmonize the postures, for example, between hip flexions.

How to reproduce this posture

Sit on the mat with your back straight. Bend your knees, lift your feet, and maintain the backs of your legs with your hands to extend your back more. Maintain this posture and keep your chest well open to improve your pulmonary capacity. Then, you can extend the legs and release your hands.

How long should you maintain this posture?

For 5–10 breaths, but it is important to keep your back straight without collapsing.

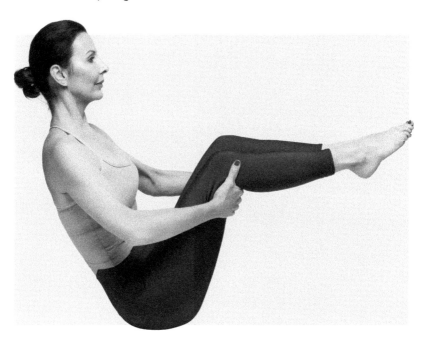

Alternatives and modifications

Keep your hands behind your legs to hold them and further extend your back.

37. Savasana - Meditation

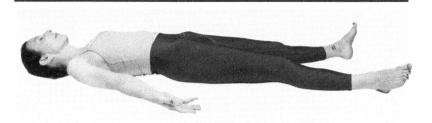

The benefits of this posture

This posture allows the body, soul, and spirit to relax. An essential phase of the practice is to recover your calm and connect with your quintessence. Use this Savasana time to practice full consciousness: take the time to integrate the thoughts that come up and let them go. Realize what you feel, then let go.

How to reproduce this posture

Lie on the ground. Turn your palms up and let the feet go down on their sides. If you are cold, cover yourself.

Alternatives and modifications for this posture

You can place a block under the bolster vertically placed on your mat, then lie on it. Having the upper body elevated can be very enjoyable. You can also place a bolster under your knees to promote relaxation. If you are pregnant, I suggest you use this Savasana position to enjoy this precious moment fully.

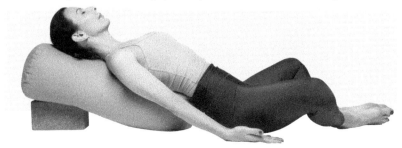

Yin Program to
Fight Anxiety

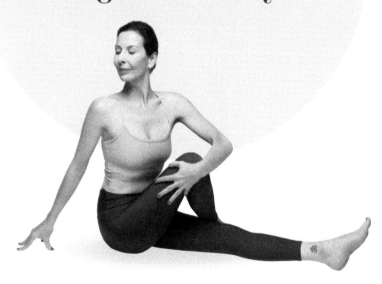

Y in Yoga and visualizations reduce stress and anxiety and contribute to your well-being. The first step is to identify your own behaviors and then it's a good idea to analyze them to understand yourself better. Write down your traumas and pain during your crises of anxiety and replace them with positive mental images that bring peace and calm to you.

It has been scientifically proven that your brain can be reprogrammed by the messages it receives. The stronger the messages and the more they are repeated, the more they direct the brain. It is thus indispensable to feel the changes you want as if they were real and to deepen them regularly.

I often notice that my clients have problems placing themselves in a state of calm, deep relaxation. Their anxiety does not allow them to relax. Even after a Ying Yoga session, they are still worried and preoccupied. This proven breathing method allows you to let go.

Pranayamas (Breathing Exercises) - *Nadi Shodana*, Alternate Nostril Breathing

Breathing is living. In the yogic tradition, breathing is the manifestation of Prana and Chi.

The word *'pranayama'* comes from the Sanskrit word Prana, meaning "life," "breath," "energy," and yama, "exercise." With alternate nostril breathing, you balance the energies between the energy canals: nadis of ida, and pingala. You harmonize Yin and Yang within your body in balance with the universe and yourself.

In our era, it seems essential to me to take the time to integrate this regular breathing exercise as it can help calm you mentally and increase your vitality. The pandemic has skyrocketed the cases of anxiety, which is another reason to integrate *Nadi Shodana* into your daily life.

In my work as a therapist, I notice that applying this breathing has precious effects. This is as true for children and teenagers as it is for adults. The results are impressive. Some finally relax and feel relative interior peace, while others liberate themselves from their state of chronic anxiety.

I had a girl following my sessions who came because she was always tired. A medical consultation revealed nothing. After a few sessions, she shared with me that she felt more alive and less exhausted. We then understood that she was suffering from chronic fatigue simply because she was not breathing correctly. Her mental state had influenced her breathing, so it became shorter and more superficial.

How to practice *Nadi Shodana*

1. Sit down comfortably with your back straight.
2. Your left palm must rest comfortably on your thigh, while your right hand is placed in front of your face. The right-hand position is called *Vishnu Mudra* in yoga.
3. Inhale deeply through your nose, then exhale.
4. Close your right nostril with your right thumb. Breath in a slow, constant manner in your left nostril.
5. At the end of the inspiration, close your left nostril with your ring finger, while freeing the right nostril.
6. Exhale through the right nostril (while keeping the left nostril closed).
7. Inhale slowly through the right nostril (while keeping the left nostril closed).
8. Close the right nostril again, open the left nostril and exhale slowly through it.

- Alternate nostril breathing balances masculine and feminine energy, the Yin and Yang.
- You benefit from more oxygen.
- Breathing increases your vitality and your life energy.
- You have more stamina and strength.
- Your creativity increases.
- Your mind calms.
- You benefit from a calm state and interior peace.
- You rebalance the breathing between your two nostrils.
- You restore the balance between your two brain hemispheres.
- You relieve stress and anxiety.
- You benefit from reduced blood pressure.
- You improve the quality of your concentration.
- You strengthen your breathing system and your lungs.
- You eliminate more toxins present inside your body.
- You clean your sinuses (good for the allergies).

I strongly recommend integrating your breathing before or after your Yin Yoga practice. You can even integrate it during moments of crisis to calm yourself without practicing postures.

Many teenagers who come to see me with chronic anxiety have practiced *Nadi Shodana* in difficult moments, and the results are very satisfying.

Breathing Is Living!

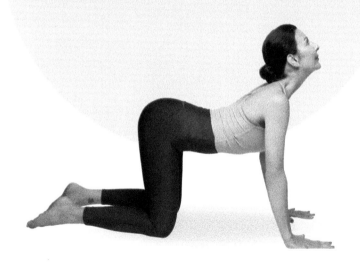

Creative Visualization:
A Different Meditation

C reative visualization is a technique that has existed for a long time. It uses mental images and your dreams to manifest thoughts in your life. You have the power to create the life you want. Before getting there, it is necessary to prepare seriously and feel things genuinely.

Many books on this subject have influenced me since my adolescence. Shakti Gawain, For instance, wrote about creative visualization and the development of intuition[3]. She helped me understand I had the power to have the life I wanted. After reading her books, creative visualization gave direction to my life.

The ability to create what I wanted with my thoughts and imagination had enormous power, and I took control of my destiny. Instead of letting myself drift about, I was aware of what I wanted and took the time to meditate on that, write about it, and imagine how I felt when I received what I wanted. It was incredible. Yes, it took some time, but my goals and desires were being realised.

Every day, I sat in front of a candle and fixated on it. It was like yoga for eyes, Trataka. In this technique, your gaze fixes on the flame, with the goal of not closing your eyes to blink. Tears often flow afterwards; it is the Trataka cleaning process for the health of your eyes.

Back then, I did not know this technique, and I used the candle only because it helped me to stay focused. It was as if keeping my gaze fixed on a stationary object encouraged my concentration on my goal and made my imagination more accessible. By practicing and learning more about the subject, I often encountered my subconscious and its importance. You are not conscious of that psychic state, but it can influence your behavior. After some brief reflection, I told myself it was better to use that in my favor.

---

3. Shakti Gawain, Creative Visualisation, Nataraj Publishing, 2002.

Do you talk to yourself? Most people's internal dialogue, spoken out loud or not, is generally negative. Please be aware that your subconscious is always listening to your internal discourse. It is essential to be mindful of the way you talk to yourself; write it down and rewrite it to create the destiny you want.

Here are some concrete examples. A long-time acquaintance often said that whatever she was doing, she always ended up without money. At first, that seemed strange to me because she and her husband earned a good living. I did not believe it and was sure she said that to attract attention and play the victim. Maybe that was what she was doing, but, indeed, she always had little money, with unexpected bills, fines, and the list went on and on. It resulted from the discourse she always had with the people around her and herself. Her subconscious was recording it, and she was receiving the energy she was sending into the universe: I don't have any money.

I have a very close friend who is always trying to lose weight. She tells everyone, including herself, that she's too fat and does not want to eat anymore. The message she transmits to her subconscious is that "I am fat and do not want to eat anymore." That brings me to the next principle of visualization: affirmations have more power than negations. The subconscious does not understand 'do not want', just the verb, in this case, the verb 'eat' and the adjective 'fat'. It is better to express the desire differently: "I am thin and beautiful. My body is beautiful. I eat healthily and take care of myself." Then you need to meditate on the topic to feel it. That will affect how you behave and improve your lifestyle, which will lead to weight loss. It goes without saying that this visualization must be done regularly to find its roots and for the person in question to believe it and, above all, feel it.

Working on what you believe and how you perceive yourself is essential. If you are convinced that you will never get money and are fat, that will not change because you are repeating that to yourself daily. It would be best if you also worked on your emotions and what you feel. Visualize your feelings when you have money in abundance. How would you behave? What would you do, etc.?

The same thing applies to my friend's case: for the creative visualization to work, she needs to believe she is thin, see herself as thin and feel how she would move with greater ease thanks to her toned body.

Believing in your goals is the base. Shouting it louder will not get you what you want; feeling it deep inside yourself will. You can influence your emotions with your words and thoughts, and vice versa. The affirmations remain an essential part of this technique, but the feeling part is also indispensable.

It is imperative, when you visualize your goals, that you remain focused. The candle technique might be useful to you. You can also carry out this creative visualization meditation in the Savasana position, the final relaxation after practicing yoga. For it to be possible for your goals to anchor and become a reality, I think it is necessary to know yourself and find moments to practice regularly. We always return to the fundamental concept of therapy: it is best to see humans as whole and link the body, spirit, and soul.

Elementary points for practicing creative visualization

- Decide when you will practice it regularly, for example, before or after your yoga practice.
- Become aware of your internal discourse.
- Put down on paper what you would like to manifest in your life.
- Write your goal and describe it positively with affirmations.
- Remove all doubts and negations that could block you.

■ Remember that the subconscious rules your behavior and take responsibility for deciding what you would like to manifest in your life.

■ Be vigilant in keeping the habit and practice the visualization like a ritual at fixed hours.

The power of thought

I would like to connect creative visualization with the power of thought and the law of attraction. Since the origins of Yin Yoga come from Taoism, I will quote Buddha: "What you have become is what you thought." Asian people have known this principle for centuries.

In my opinion, we are focused on technological progress in our society, and we lose the connection with our intuition bit by bit. What Buddha said seems so simple and logical to me. Why not integrate it into our lives? Why is there so much suffering when we do not get what we want? Why are we not satisfied with the person we have become? The answer is simple: we have lost awareness of the power of our thoughts and let ourselves live without taking responsibility for what is happening to us.

I observed that frequently during my professional work. When I asked the clients what they wanted to manifest in their lives, their answers were often opposite to my request; they told me what they did not want. When I pointed out that that was not what I wanted to know, they were unhappy, to say the least. Their anger often related to their belated understanding that they did not really know what they wanted—but it was initially aimed at me. Then, sometimes, there was some introspection, which led them to understand what they wanted in life. Generally, there were changes in their daily lives and significant personal development.

Since every change demands some effort and can be scary, this is not obvious. The question was then to know if they preferred to live in situations of little authenticity that they'd acquired, or if they would make the effort to be responsible for their lives and begin to make changes to manifest what they really wanted.

Your thoughts become words, words convert into gestures, gestures form your character, and your character represents your personality and destiny.

That sentence illustrates the importance of thoughts, the origin of creative vision. You first need to decide what you want, then you need to express and feel it clearly, so it becomes a reality.

The Law of Attraction

The law of attraction is a universal principle, like the law of gravity. It is based on the principle that your thoughts and your emotional state have vibrations and that you attract the same energies you emit.

AS A HUMAN BEING YOU CONSTANTLY SPREAD ENERGY OUT INTO THE UNIVERSE. WHEN YOU ARE HAPPY AND CONTENT, YOU ATTRACT THE SAME FREQUENCY.

The best example is the radio: if you switch on 101.1 on FM1, you cannot receive 99.2 on FM2. It's the same with vibrations.

Have you ever noticed that when you are feeling good, only positive things happen to you? Then, when something happens to change your mood, your vibrations are no longer the same. The sequence of adverse events continues if you fail to change your vibrations. It is thus crucial to learn how to change your feelings to manifest what you want.

In my therapeutic practice, I see about fifteen people daily and am constantly surprised by their energy, which I feel powerfully. Some of those vibrations are not positive. As a result, I need to work seriously on myself and my emotional state so that the energy of others does not invade me.

I also decided to feel right! I thought long and hard about escaping my vicious cycle of negative emotions. I found a method that works very well and would like to share it, so that you, too, can take responsibility for your life and manifest what you want. Choose a moment in your day and write down or repeat all the things you appreciate in your life. The gratefulness you'll feel will have extremely positive vibrations. You will feel deep well-being that will attract vibrations of the same frequency. You will not only attract things you would like but also benefit from a calm state of mind. It's a simple and efficient principle. The lists below of positive and negative emotions to help you change your vibrations.

Positive Vibrations

- Joy
- Gratitude
- Pride
- Love
- Friendship
- Trust
- A general positive attitude.

Negative Vibrations

- Jealousy
- Disappointment
- Mistrust
- Confusion
- Solitude
- Sadness
- Envy.

- Think about what you want to attract and manifest in your life.
- Write your goals on paper to remove potential negative language. The subconscious is as powerful as creative visualization.
- Take responsibility for your life.
- Use gratitude and emotions with positive vibrations to change your mindset.
- Repeat and visualize your goals daily so they can anchor within you and become a reality.

Karma

Do you remember that Yin Yoga origins from Taoism, and that one of its three pillars is Buddhism?

The karma principle is the central dogma in Buddhism. Your actions determine how you feel and what happens to you in the present. Using the law of attraction as a basis, that means your actions have vibrations attracting similar vibrations.

The karma law is often misinterpreted: if you act generously, the people who benefit must repay you. That conception is weak and does not correspond to the nature of karma. When you act ethically, it fills you with joy, which results in positive vibrations and a feeling of deep well-being. You then attract vibrations of the same frequency.

The belief in and the application of those laws of karma and attraction contribute to a more significant vibration. Your goals manifest, and you become a better version of yourself.

Therapeutic Visualization

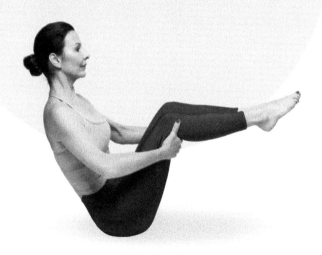

n psychoneuroimmunology, visualization is frequently used with meditation, hypnosis, and biofeedback. Scientific research has proven its efficiency.

In my work as a therapist, I often refer to my clients' internal and external resources. The internal mental resources, resilience, and the ability to imagine the goals are set in motion with this technique. Therapeutic creative visualization changes the mental imagery and thus the emotional state, which has a repercussion on the body's felt emotions.

You learn to replace sensations of physical and psychological pain (like anxiety) to treat traumatic events. You visualize images of mental and physical well-being from that perspective. You use your intuition and your subconscious. Your internal voice.

How to practice therapeutic visualization

To access to your intuition, practicing Yin Yoga is essential for placing yourself in a calm state. Then, you are ready to go through various steps.

1. Create an image, a general and concrete visualization, by closing your eyes.

2. Deepen your understanding by repeating it regularly and adding details to bring it to life.

3. Analyze your visualization, and remove any possible blockages, negations, and counterproductive beliefs anchored in you. Reformulate them with affirmations. Sometimes, writing things down can be helpful. Writing and talking to your therapist often helps you to notice what is rooted inside you. You can then access your subconscious and realize what is really happening inside your mind.

4. Continue to visualize daily and feel you are becoming autonomous; you are mastering your mental images. You strengthen your self-healing abilities because you feel the

created mental image manifesting in each of your cells. Your mental and physical attitudes have changed. It is necessary to continue this visualization so it can anchor deeply in your being.

As you can see, this technique acts to change behaviors and reduce stress. I often use it to work on addiction problems and help some clients control their exam stress, for example.

Therapeutic visualization has been proven effective in treating the following:

- Depression
- Anxiety
- Chronic back pain
- Arthritis
- Motor functions
- Fibromyalgia
- Osteoporosis and osteoarthritis
- Nightmares
- Stress-related stomach pain
- Consequences of chemotherapy.

Body, mind, and spirit work in synergy to reach your goals.

In case you are still skeptical, here's an example to illustrate your mental power. It has been demonstrated that virtual training has the same impact as real training. Do you realize that imagining and making an effort has the potential to create muscular mass? I think it is necessary to be aware of that and to learn how to use it. Performance visualizations have been part of sports and physical re-education programs for a long time. Obviously, some pathologies mentioned above are often treated by traditional medical methods, the mental imagery is complementary.

I invite you to take a moment for some introspection: what preoccupies you and causes you to worry? Write your visualization while respecting therapeutic visualization's four steps. Practice visualization regularly after a Yin Yoga session. Take the time to write down your concern to understand; replace the blockages by rewriting them with affirmations. Remember that treating your hardships with your mind, body, and spirit yields better results.

Conclusion

Seeing your troubles as messages and progressing along the self-healing path while considering your body, spirit, and mind allows you to deepen your self-knowledge and respond to what upsets you. It's best to take responsibility for your life. It seems so easy to blame others or external circumstances. However, it is critical to understand that the pain linked to your mindset has enormous power.

In our performance-oriented society, physical effort and exercises play an essential role. Yes, it is crucial to let the energy flow in every sense of the term. However, I am amazed to see how mental aspects are pushed aside. You have the power to create the life you want, and your ailments tell you what obstacles to overcome. Often, exterior distractions prevent you from remaining connected with your quintessence. A lack of trust leads you to delegate the responsibility to others, like the doctor, who certainly seems to know what to do.

You are a whole being in which mind, body, and spirit, are linked. Live with full awareness and listen to your body to interpret its messages so you can live in perfect health.

Stress and anxiety are ailments of our current society. If you add a lack of physical activity and recurring ailments like back, hip or shoulder pain, etc., you can understand how essential it is to adopt some movements integrating the mind-body connection. You will then experience the benefit of that integration in your daily life. That is why I suggest Yin, a yoga discipline accessible to everyone! During this practice, postures are maintained for many minutes to allow the mind to calm. You will also discover a particular meditation, creative visualization (how to reprogram your subconscious) to integrate your mind, body, and spirit.

This book is a detailed guide to practicing Yin Yoga with

complete autonomy. Access to its benefits is provided via many
elegant Yin explanations.

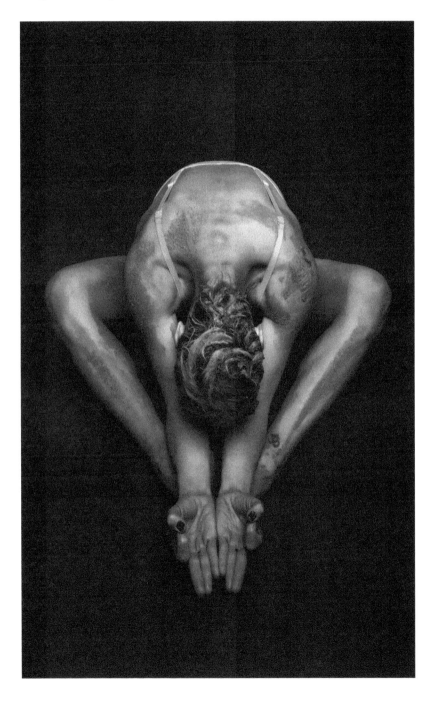